Yamamoto

Managing Hospitals

SHELDON ROVIN
LOIS GINSBERG

EDITORS

Managing Hospitals

LESSONS FROM THE
JOHNSON & JOHNSON–
WHARTON FELLOWS PROGRAM
IN MANAGEMENT
FOR NURSES

Jossey-Bass Publishers • San Francisco

MANAGING HOSPITALS
Lessons from the Johnson & Johnson–Wharton Fellows Program in Management for Nurses
by Sheldon Rovin and Lois Ginsberg, Editors

Copyright © 1991 by: Jossey-Bass Inc., Publishers
350 Sansome Street
San Francisco, California 94104

Library of Congress Cataloging-in-Publication Data

Managing hospitals : lessons from the Johnson & Johnson–Wharton
  Fellows Program in Management for Nurses / Sheldon Rovin, Lois
  Ginsberg, editors. — 1st ed.
      p.   cm. — (The Jossey-Bass health series)
  Includes bibliographical references and index.
  ISBN 1-55542-380-9
    1. Nursing services — Administration.   2. Nurse administrators.
I. Rovin, Sheldon.   II. Ginsberg, Lois, date.   III. Johnson &
Johnson–Wharton Fellows Program in Management for Nurses.
IV. Series.
    [DNLM: 1. Hospital Administration — United States.   2. Hospital
Planning — United States.   3. Nursing Services — organization &
administration — United States.   WX 150 M2667]
RT89.M3844 1991
362.1'1'068 — dc20
DNLM/DLC
for Library of Congress   91-7087
                                                                        CIP

The Wandel and Hershey material abstracted in Chapter Six is used with
the permission of *Omega: The International Journal of Management Science.*

Manufactured in the United States of America. Nearly all Jossey-Bass
books and jackets are printed on recycled paper that contains at least
50 percent recycled waste, including 10 percent postconsumer waste.
Many of our materials are also printed with vegetable-based ink; during
the printing process these inks emit fewer volatile organic compounds
(VOCs) than petroleum-based inks. VOCs contribute to the formation of
smog.

JACKET DESIGN BY WILLI BAUM

FIRST EDITION

HB Printing   10 9 8 7 6 5 4 3 2

Code 9181

The Jossey-Bass Health Series

Contents

Preface

The impetus that gave rise to the Johnson & Johnson–Wharton Fellows Program in Management for Nurses is the need for top-level nurse executives to understand and use the theory and practical skills of management so they can help lead their hospitals into an increasingly uncertain future by design rather than reaction. It is also the stimulus for writing this book. But this book is not the story of the Johnson & Johnson–Wharton Fellows Program; it is an outcome of the program. It presents the learnings of the participants and faculty of the program.

The ten chapters that constitute this book represent the learnings of nine years of programs and experiences with 357 of the top nursing executive leaders (fellows) throughout the United States and in several other countries. A brief description of some of the program's features may enable those unfamiliar with it to understand how it gave rise to this book. Selected competitively, the fellows must, as a condition of acceptance, demonstrate the support of their hospitals by securing the agreement of their CEOs or COOs to spend the last two and one-half days of the program at the University of Pennsylvania with them, planning how to bring some of the learnings back to their hospitals. This is one of the unique features of the program; another is the networking that occurs not only during the three-week program but throughout the year in the form of a quarterly newsletter, as well as at a yearly advanced management education conference when the fellows return to Philadelphia.

In the beginning, after a survey of hospital leaders and Wharton faculty for curriculum suggestions, a program was designed to encompass the management information, skills, and controversies that seemed most challenging and relevant. As anyone who has participated in an adult education experience knows, however, the range of material absorbed extends far beyond the classroom: learning from the other participants is at least as valuable as the formal lectures (and goes on into the early hours of many mornings and on weekends). Not being particularly reticent (an understatement), each group of nurse fellows has let us know what about the program was worthwhile and what needed to be changed, updated, added, or eliminated. The COOs and CEOs have done so as well. As a result, the curriculum over the years has managed to be current and responsive to need. There is no doubt, however, that the teaching and the learning have always gone both ways: the fellows have taught the faculty as much as the faculty have taught them.

When we first contemplated a book based on the curriculum of the Johnson & Johnson–Wharton Fellows Program, it seemed an easy task to communicate in print what was so exciting in the classroom. It is apparent to us, however, that no matter how useful and interesting the subject matter, it is the exchange among participants and with faculty over the subject matter that makes adult learning so stimulating and productive — and different from most other formal education. This exchange is the most difficult element to convey in a book. But part of what makes the program unique is the opportunity for participants to spend large, uninterrupted blocks of time learning, interacting, evaluating, reflecting, and challenging.

Over the years, fellows who started out as directors of nursing (the title changes are fascinating evidence of the change in the role and recognition of nurse executives) have become vice presidents of patient-care services, administrators of many areas of the hospital, and COOs and CEOs. It has become clear that the leadership and management skills that are the focus of the Wharton Fellows Program are necessary to survive in any and all of these positions. The management subjects described in the following chapters are important not only for nurse managers but for administrators, pharmacy directors, physician managers, allied health professionals, and, indeed, for anyone having to manage resources in a health care setting.

This book has two central themes: understanding and organizational learning. Because of the frenetic nature of managerial life in hospitals, managers tend to be concerned with getting things done—what to do and how to do it. If they understand why things work or do not work, so much the better, but understanding is secondary. The modus operandi is to get the job done or solve the problem and get on to something else. That attitude may work in the short run, but in the long run it is a conduit to disaster. More than anything else, long-term organizational health depends on understanding, knowing why the unit or service or hospital succeeds or fails, and why the stakeholders act as they do. And though we devote much of the book to what has to be done and how to do it, more of the writing is aimed at understanding what we do and how we do it, as well as the reasons behind decisions and what makes them sound.

The second theme is learning about our organizations. *Organizational learning* means understanding the organization, its people, practices, and culture. The organization that has the capacity to learn, and to adjust and change as a result, has a real advantage. But organizational learning is not individual learning; it is individuals learning collectively. It requires understanding the assumptions, particularly the implicit ones, that guide organizational behavior. Obviously, organizations do not behave; people behave. But when people behave—for example, cooperatively and interdependently—the organization takes on the cast of that behavior. And, conversely, when people behave uncooperatively and independent of the organization's goals, the organization assumes a form corresponding to that behavior.

When organizational learning occurs, decisions are not made in a vacuum; people at all levels understand them and the goals that give rise to them. Organizational learning enables decision making and behavior to be generally reproduced at the various levels, and it makes the achievement of goals more likely as a consequence. Organizational learning is what makes it possible for an organization to become coordinated, integrated, and harmonious.

This book is a management book. It is for executives who manage in clinical settings, but it is not about clinical practice. Both science and art undergird management, just as both science and art support clinical nursing. Although clinical examples are given, they are used only to make points and elucidate how management information can be applied or understood. Most of the authors of the chapters are business school faculty members who, by dint of their experience with medical care administrators and institutions both in the classroom and as on-site consultants, bring the fruits of their background and work to bear on medical care management issues. A premise of this book is that there are management concepts and precepts that have universal application in any business or organization. Their application to medical care organizations is, we believe, salutary and desirable.

Overview of the Contents

We have organized this book to represent the flow of the curriculum used in the Wharton Fellows Program. It has three parts: "Managing the Planning Process," "Economic Issues and Support Systems," and "People Skills and Managing Behavior." We believe that these represent the essentials of management, whether the organization is small or large, rural or urban, or for-profit or not-for-profit. Planning gives us direction, function, and design. Economics and support systems help us apply the resources of money and information. Behavior — that of others and ourselves — determines the quality of implementation. And how well we manage all three components in the aggregate determines the quality of what is done and the work lives of those who do it.

Part One covers planning and its connections to marketing and organizational design. Chapter One makes a case for planning as the manager's main work: an ongoing, participatory process that is a fundamental part of directing the organization toward achieving its goals. Chapter Two demystifies marketing by treating it as a part of the planning process, showing how marketing methods are a legitimate means of furthering the purpose of the organization if used properly. Chapter Three explains how to think about linking structure to purpose.

Part Two deals with two of the most important resources available to health care managers: money and information. Chapter Four argues that economic analysis should contribute to decision making if it is to be effective. Although the emphasis is never on saving money to the detriment of quality care, considerations of cost and benefit, and risk, must be included. Chapter Five provides a framework for understanding financial issues. As part of being able to analyze cost factors and understand the financial implications of decisions, managers must have a grasp of the fundamentals of financial management. Chapter Six explains how to use decision making as a tool for planning—for analyzing staffing, costs, inventory, and other management areas. Operations research provides a methodology for decision making by thinking in terms of models and testing. Finally, the growing importance of information systems in the management of both central and departmental information is explored in Chapter Seven. This chapter stresses that information technology must serve managers' needs, not the other way around.

Part Three recognizes that the most important aspects of management in any organization concern the individuals and their ability to work with one another. Chapter Eight approaches the issue of managing people from the point of view of one person dealing with another: How do you get someone to actually do what you want him or her to do? Chapter Nine addresses the quality of managers' relationships to one another: How do you clarify responsibility and roles, and how do you integrate people needs and work needs? Finally, Chapter Ten suggests some productive approaches for handling conflict and change. Negotiation as a methodology is explored as a framework for taking a fresh look at human encounters that affect work and the organization.

In sum, we want to suggest a way of using this book that will facilitate learning and application. Our suggestion is born of experience with the program. It is, simply, to read and think in groups about the ideas and tools described, rather than or in addition to doing so individually. We know that when more than one person from a unit or organization reads about the same idea and discusses it and understands it, the likelihood of its acceptance and application is enhanced. Our suggestion is to organize a special dialogue around the ideas that interest you or to discuss them at scheduled meetings. Try some of the ideas, play with them, change them, and turn them into instruments of your own—but do so collectively. We do this in groups of forty at the University of Pennsylvania, our place of business. We believe you can do the same at your own place of business.

Acknowledgments

Because this book is an outgrowth of the Johnson & Johnson–Wharton Fellows Program, we would like to acknowledge the people responsible for seeing that the program remains innovative and relevant to the needs of health care management. We start by acknowledging the Johnson & Johnson Family of Companies Contributions Fund, whose continuing sponsorship of the program contains only one stipulation—that the program be the best we can make it. Philip Doyle and Curtis Weeden have skillfully and lovingly steered the fellows program for Johnson & Johnson since its inception. Victoria Strohmeyer, also from Johnson & Johnson, for the past three years has been instrumental to the program's continuing success. The members of the advisory committee have faithfully contributed not only their time and professional judgment, but their originality, ideas, and support to both the fellows and us. In particular, we cannot give enough credit or thanks to Dorothy del Bueno, Robert Cathcart, Claire Fagin, Thomas Gilmore, and William Pierskalla, who have been with the program from the beginning, as well as to the fellows who served on the committee as representatives of their classes. We are especially grateful to all the faculty, who have looked forward each year to a new class of fellows and who, by their expertise, enthusiasm, and teaching skill, have made the program what it is. The value added by the talent and devotion of Claudine Greene, the program coordinator, cannot be overstated. Our good fortune in having a superb and patient editor, Tobia L. Worth, has made it possible for us to see this book through to completion.

In the initial design of this book, it was our intention to

include in each chapter original case material, to be provided by the Johnson & Johnson–Wharton fellows based on their own experiences. There is no doubt in our minds that if we had been able to do this, the book would have been better for it. However, due to publishing and other constraints, it was decided to leave this material out of the book. Nevertheless, the faculty were able to use the fellows' analyses to inform their chapters as well as their teaching. We want to thank the following Johnson & Johnson–Wharton fellows for providing cases that were thoughtful, provocative, and instructive: Ann Ameigh, vice president of nursing, Geisinger Medical Center, Danville, Pennsylvania; Doris Armstrong, vice president of nursing, Hartford Hospital, Hartford, Connecticut; Mary Butler, vice president of patient services, Sacred Heart Medical Center, Spokane, Washington; Beryl Chickerella, senior vice president of nursing, Doctors Hospital, Columbus, Ohio; Susan Crissman, senior vice president, Memorial Hospital, South Bend, Indiana; Dorothy Deremo, vice president of nursing, Henry Ford Hospital, Detroit, Michigan; Maryann Fralic, senior vice president of nursing, Robert Wood Johnson University Hospital, New Brunswick, New Jersey; Patricia Kuykendall, vice president, University of Texas Medical Branch, Galveston, Texas; Judith Murray, senior vice president of nursing service, Jewish Hospital of Cincinnati, Cincinnati, Ohio; Anne Sheetz, Massachusetts Department of Public Health, Boston; and Margaret Vosburgh, vice president of nursing services, Hoag Memorial Hospital, Newport Beach, California.

Finally, and most important, we thank the nurse executives who are the Johnson & Johnson–Wharton fellows. They have inspired all of us with their professional abilities and their personal commitment to both providers and recipients of health care. This book is dedicated to them, and to their colleagues whom we have yet to meet.

Philadelphia, Pennsylvania   Sheldon Rovin
August 1991   Lois Ginsberg

The Editors

Sheldon Rovin is professor and chairperson of the Department of Dental Care Systems, School of Dental Medicine, and professor of health care systems at the Wharton School, University of Pennsylvania. He serves as the associate director of the Leonard Davis Institute of Health Economics and director of both the Johnson & Johnson–Wharton Fellows Program in Management for Nurses and the SmithKline Beecham Executive Management Program for Directors of Hospital Pharmacy. Dr. Rovin received his D.D.S. degree (1957) and his M.S. degree (1960) from the University of Michigan. His teaching and consulting interests include planning, management development, creativity, and organizational communications. He has won several teaching awards. His publication record includes over eighty journal articles and book chapters, and he has authored or coauthored the following five books: *Oral Cancer: Detection and Diagnosis* (1973, 2nd ed.); *Individualized Instruction in a Flexible Dental Curriculum* (1973, with Timothy Smith and Elizabeth Haley); *The Programmed Textbook of Oral Pathology* (1974, with William R. Sabes and Robert M. Howell); *The Tooth Robbers: A Pro-Fluoridation Handbook* (1981, with Stephen Barrett); and *Managed Health Care and Practice Management* (1990, with Cecile A. Feldman and Laurence Brody). Prior to joining the faculty of the University of Pennsylvania, Rovin was in the inaugural class of the VA Administrative Scholars Program and dean of the School of Dentistry at the University of Washington.

Lois Ginsberg is associate director of "The Dynamics of Organization," a graduate program for mid- to upper-level managers and professionals based at the University of Pennsylvania's Graduate School of Arts and Sciences. She received her B.A. degree (1958) from the University of Michigan and then attended New York University's School of Law. Ginsberg was associate director of the Johnson & Johnson–Wharton Fellows Program from 1983 to 1990 while managing the Leonard Davis Institute's advanced education programs. Earlier, from 1976 to 1982, she was a research manager for several large social science research projects at the University of Pennsylvania.

The Contributors

Elizabeth F. Dunn is director of market development at the Thomas Jefferson University Hospital. She is an adjunct associate professor of marketing strategy at the Wharton School, where she took a postdoctorate in marketing. Dunn received her B.A. degree (1969) from Pennsylvania State University and her Ph.D. degree (1977) from Temple University in educational psychology. She has written on marketing for health educators and on physician practice enhancement.

Charles E. Dwyer is associate professor in the Graduate School of Education, University of Pennsylvania. His current research interests are in the areas of decision making, managing people, time management, and value systems. Dwyer received his M.S. degree (1962) in industrial relations and organizational behavior and his Ph.D. degree (1966) in philosophy and education from Cornell University. He is an experienced consultant and educator, his clients including General Electric, the New York Stock Exchange, Polaroid, Texaco, IBM, Xerox, AT&T, and R.J.R. Nabisco. He is the founder and chairman of the board of the Swarthmore Academy. He also chairs the Educational Leadership Division at the Graduate School of Education.

John M. Eisenberg is Sol Katz Professor of General Internal Medicine and chief of section of general internal medicine at the University of Pennsylvania. He is a graduate of Princeton University and the Washington University School of Medicine, St. Louis, Missouri. Eisenberg was a Robert Wood Johnson Foundation Clinical Scholar and earned an M.B.A. degree (1976) at the Wharton School. He is a senior fellow of the University of Pennsylvania's Leonard Davis Institute of Health Economics and has published over 140 articles and chapters on such topics as physicians' economics. His book *Doctors' Decisions and the Cost of Medical Care* was published by the Health Administration Press in 1986.

Cecile A. Feldman is associate professor of general and hospital dentistry and director for information services and quality assurance at the University of Medicine and Dentistry of New Jersey and is adjunct assistant professor of dental care systems at the University of Pennsylvania School of Dental Medicine. She received her B.A. degree (1980) in economics from the University of Pennsylvania, her D.M.D. degree (1984) from the University of Pennsylvania School of Dental Medicine, and her M.B.A. degree (1985) from the Wharton School. Her research interests include information technology, quality assurance, and cost-effectiveness. She is the author of several articles and a book, *Managed Health Care and Practice Management* (1990, with Sheldon Rovin and Laurence Brody). She is presently directing the development and implementation of a new management information system at the New Jersey Dental School. She is also a senior fellow at the Leonard Davis Institute of Health Economics. Previously, Feldman worked for the University of Pennsylvania's Planning Office and the Higher Education Finance Research Institute, where she developed numerous computerized simulation models for long-range planning.

Steven A. Finkler is professor of public and health administration, accounting, and financial management at New York University's Robert F. Wagner Graduate School of Public Service. His research includes studies on the cost-effectiveness of shortened length of hospital stay with nurse specialist follow-up. He received his B.S. degree (1971) in economics and his M.S.

degree (1972) in accounting from the Wharton School, and both his M.A. degree (1976) in economics and his Ph.D. degree (1978) in business administration from Stanford University. He is the author of *The Complete Guide to Finance and Accounting for Non-Financial Managers* (1983) and *Budgeting Concepts for Nurse Managers* (1991, second edition). Also among Dr. Finkler's publications are articles in the *New England Journal of Medicine*, the *Journal of Nursing Administration*, *Nursing Economics*, and *Health Services Research*.

Thomas North Gilmore is vice president of the Wharton Center for Applied Research, a private consulting firm that operates in cooperation with the Wharton School. He is a senior fellow at the Leonard Davis Institute of Health Economics and an adjunct professor of health care systems. He received his B.A. degree (1966) from Harvard University and his M.Arch. degree (1970) from the University of Pennsylvania. Gilmore's research and consulting focus on organizational change and interorganizational behavior and strategy. His book *Making a Leadership Change: How Organizations and Leaders Can Handle Leadership Transitions Successfully* (1988) addresses how leaders and organizations manage transitions.

John C. Hershey is professor and chair of the Department of Decision Sciences at the Wharton School and director of research for the Leonard Davis Institute of Health Economics. He received his B.S. degree (1965) from Carnegie-Mellon University in mathematics. He received both his M.S. degree (1970) in operations research and his Ph.D. degree (1970) in management science from Stanford University. His research interests include the application of operations research and decision sciences to health services delivery problems. Among his publications are articles in *Management Science, Operations Research,* and *Health Services Research.*

Lawrence G. Hrebiniak is associate professor of management at the Wharton School. He received his A.B. degree (1964) from Cornell University in economics and his M.B.A. degree

(1967) and Ph.D. degree (1971) from the State University of New York, Buffalo, in organizational theory and management. He has had considerable consulting experience in both the private and public sectors and has authored many articles for professional journals. His latest books are *Complex Organizations* (1978) and *Implementing Strategy* (1984, with William F. Joyce), which focuses on organizational design and planning decisions in the formulation and implementation of strategy.

Gregory P. Shea is senior fellow at the Leonard Davis Institute of Health Economics, a partner in the Coxe Group, which specializes in organizational issues particularly for design firms, an adjunct professor in the management department of the Wharton School and the Aresty Institute for Executive Education, and senior consultant with the Wharton Center. Shea received his M.Sc. degree (1976) from the London School of Economics in management studies and his Ph.D. degree (1981) from Yale University in administrative science. His research and consulting interests are in management of conflict and determinants of effectiveness in groups.

Mary Kaye Willian is senior clinical researcher at Mathematica Policy Research, Inc., and an adjunct assistant professor at the University of Pennsylvania School of Nursing and School of Medicine. She received her B.S. degree (1968) and M.S. degree (1973) from Indiana University School of Nursing and her M.P.H. degree (1979) and Dr. P.H. degree (1982) from the Johns Hopkins University School of Public Health. Willian was cofounder of the journal *Nursing Economics,* director of clinical economics at the Philadelphia Association for Clinical Trials, senior health policy analyst with the Medicare Prospective Payment Assessment Commission, and senior health planner with the Maryland Health Planning Commission. She was selected as one of the Outstanding Young Women of America in 1982.

Managing Hospitals

PART 1

Managing
the Planning Process

CHAPTER 1

The Process of Planning

Sheldon Rovin

This chapter is called "The Process of Planning" because planning is a never-ending process. It is or should be the main business of executives, be they vice presidents of nursing or CEOs or any manager responsible for how things turn out. Planning both has and gives purpose. One purpose of planning is to make plans, not to come up with A Plan. Another is to unleash and capitalize on the creativity that resides in the people of your organization. Still another is to provide an enabling mechanism to question the assumptions on which all previous plans are based. Planning leads to the exploration of possibilities for your organization in a way that marshals the efforts of the people who work in it in a common direction: It gives purpose.

If you are looking for a planning model that is a step-by-step, linear progression that leaves you with a plan, stop reading! Instead, go to the nearest management book, look up planning in the index, find the indicated page, and you will see a planning model that looks something like Figure 1.1 or Figure 1.2.

The planning model in Figure 1.1 seldom, if ever, is effective. It is too complicated, too much dependent on data gathering, and too little dependent on ideas, creativity, and the involvement of people. Something just as ineffective, but much closer to the actual planning that goes on in many hospitals,

Figure 1.1. Typical Planning Model.

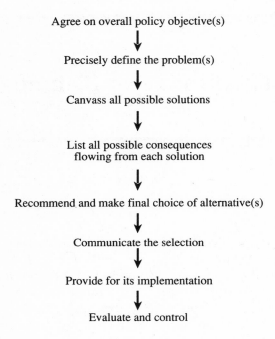

Agree on overall policy objective(s)

Precisely define the problem(s)

Canvass all possible solutions

List all possible consequences
flowing from each solution

Recommend and make final choice of alternative(s)

Communicate the selection

Provide for its implementation

Evaluate and control

is displayed in Figure 1.2. As can be seen by the huge gap between intended and actual outcomes, it does not get you where you want to go.

The reasons for these drawbacks of linear planning are simple: Implementers are seldom involved in the planning, and typical planning is riddled with concerns for problem solving, focusing on answers rather than questions.

Most organizations are where they are because of the way they have met the various crises that came along. This means that they are where they are more by chance than by design. The planning process I focus on in this chapter gets you closer to where you really want to go, not by neglecting crises, which you cannot do, but by enabling you to deal with crises in the much larger context of your goals—that is, what you want to do. Putting it another way, the organization gets where it is more by design than by chance. This planning process is called *interactive planning,* and it was developed by Russell Ackoff (1981).

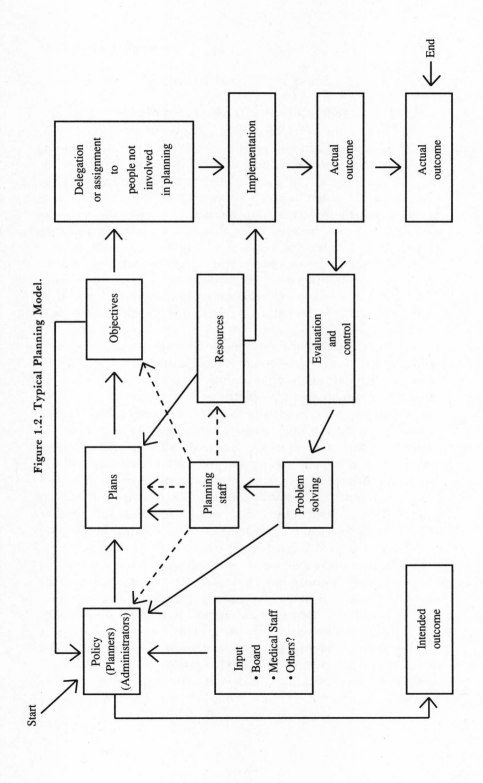

Figure 1.2. Typical Planning Model.

Flaws of Typical Planning

Typical planning is flawed in several of the following ways:

1. Planning is usually done by parts of an organization rather than the organization as a whole. As a result, planning generally consists of problems to solve or wants generated by the administration or an individual department independent of the rest of the organization. When the issue is an administrative one, it usually stems from a crisis or a reaction to a competitor, or it may be a result of the administration's acceding to pressure from a unit. When the issue arises from a department, it is a request to fix something, to get more of something, or to start something new. Regardless of its origin, the issue is seldom subjected to deliberation by the organization's other units, even those expected to do the implementation or that will be influenced by it.

This type of planning denies the principle that an organization such as a hospital is more than the sum of its parts. Planning for each part of an organization independently of the others does not eliminate most problems or lead to generally satisfying outcomes. A system (organization) that works well is more a function of the interaction or relationship of its parts than the individual parts themselves. An organization's problems come chiefly from interaction of its parts (departments), particularly the competition for resources among them, than from within the departments. A hospital, for example, may have the finest surgery department in the land, but at a cost inimical to other departments that could provide a better market for the hospital and a more needed service for its customers — that is, patients. The whole of an organization is much more than the sum of its parts, and planning for the organization as a whole is at its most effective only when the parts participate.

2. A second flaw is equating problem solving with planning. Problem solving usually means correcting deficiencies or getting rid of something you do not want. Nobody, with the possible exception of consultants, wants problems. However, getting rid of something you do not want does not guarantee you anything better. Witness what happens when you change

channels on your television set because the program is lousy. Closer to home, replacing a poorly performing department head does not mean you will automatically get someone better. Nor does replacing one ineffective computerized information system with another guarantee anything better. The idea of planning is to make your organization better, not keep it the same. Even if you solve the problem, you only end up in the same place you were before the problem appeared. And that same solution frequently causes other problems.

3. Forecasting is considered an integral part of planning. A great deal of the present is wasted on attempts to forecast the future (Ackoff, 1986). About the only thing managers can predict accurately is that the unexpected will happen. What appears clear and predictable on paper turns out, too often, to be muddy and notably different than expected in actuality. Managers cannot forecast what the actual demands will be for just one work day, so how can they predict accurately what is going to happen to a hospital — an organization with thousands of people — months or years ahead?

Physical phenomena such as the weather can be forecast somewhat. But anything influenced by the behavior of people, such as organizations and government, cannot be predicted accurately. The economic, political, and social universe in which hospitals operate is affected more by human behavior than by physical events. Project yourselves back ten years. Who could have foretold that health care would be treated as an economic commodity? Who could have predicted prospective reimbursement and DRGs, hospitals competing (for patients) no differently from other businesses, and hospitals turning away patients for inability to pay? Who could have predicted that hundreds of hospitals would close?

Most forecasting is extrapolation of past experience into the future. However, ways of doing things in the past work for the future only so long as the pattern of the future mimics that of the past. But now the rate of change of information and technology has decreased the effectiveness of using past experience to make projections of the future (Toffler, 1971; Drucker, 1969).

The aim is to reduce the need to forecast by controlling

more of what we do (Ackoff, 1986). The future depends more
on what happens between now and then. This means it depends
on decisions still to be made.

4. A fourth flaw of typical planning is its external focus.
Strategic planning is out of vogue now (Hurst, 1986). It does
not work well and probably never had a chance to work well
because the method focuses largely on the organization's external environment, whereas most of its control is internal. The
difference between success and failure of an organization is internal: what the people of your organization value, believe, and
do. Internal strength succeeds even in the face of extraordinary
external turbulence because knowing who you are, what you
can do, and what you cannot do gives the organization the confidence and stability to know when to adapt to an external stimulus (opportunity or threat) or not. A part of planning is understanding the internal strengths and weaknesses of your internal
environment well enough to know whether to respond to an external environmental stimulus and how to respond if you should
choose to do so.

5. Typical planning is associated with gathering huge
amounts of data to support the thrusts the organization wants
to make. Extraordinary amounts of time are spent gathering
data, many of which are not germane to the decision at hand.
The important planning decisions made at an organizationwide
level can seldom wait until the relevant information deemed
necessary to make a safe, low-risk decision is available. Decisions that distinguish your organization from another, the ones
that make the difference in whether your organization succeeds
or fails, cannot wait for a complete environmental analysis and
a thorough knowledge of likely outcomes. As a general rule,
the more data or information you have or gather about a decision, the less important the decision. (See "Environmental Analysis," below.)

6. A final flaw overlaps some of the others, but it is distinct
and important enough to merit discussion. Namely, planning
typically relies almost exclusively on left-brain activity. Analytical models, forecasting methods, data collection, quantifica-
tion, and logic are the most frequently employed tools of plan-

ning. Intuition and imagination ordinarily are not thought of as part of the repertoire of the planner. Yet imagination and intuition (making leaps of insight from "incomplete" knowledge or from feelings), along with other right-brain functions such as synthesis (putting pieces together to make wholes) and the ability to envisage relationships among sometimes quite disparate functions, are more valuable to planning, particularly when the aim is to set your hospital apart from others.

This is not to denigrate the left-brain functions of logic and analysis; the object is to elevate the right-brain functions of imagination and intuition at least to an equal footing — in other words, to achieve an integration of both functions.

Language of Planning

There is little value in trying to define planning. Arguably, this flies in the face of fulfilling my academic destiny, that is, using definitions and other conveyances to categorize and place concepts in neat niches. But to define planning would give it a static dimension contrary to the fluidity and changing nature of what effective planning is all about. Instead, the nature of planning can be expressed better by the words used to describe it. Words such as *values, mission,* and *participation.* Words such as *continuous planning, client focus, risk taking,* and *abandonment* are used. And still other words that describe the process are *trying things, experimentation, measurement,* and *learning.* Some of these words are explained below, and others later in the context of their use.

Values. Identifying *values,* particularly a set of values shared by the people of your organization, is the foundation of planning. What you stand for as an organization and as individuals constitutes the organization, and the way in which your values coincide with those of the people you serve must be identified, made legitimate through consensus, and shared with all the stakeholders in your organization.

Mission is the embodiment of your organization's values. Mission statements are written expressions of these values. Mission statements include goals and objectives. Goals are what you want to be and objectives are what you have to achieve in order to be what you want to be. This is discussed in detail in a later section on mission statements.

It is through *participation* that consensus is reached, commitment occurs, and implementation improves. Participation is the immediate and most lasting benefit of planning. Participation is enabling. Participants learn how decisions are made, how others think, and what difficulties others experience. Participation enhances the quality of work life, makes people feel good about their organization, and gives people at least some control over what happens in their work. It gives people ownership—a real stake in the organization and its outcomes.

Truly effective implementation requires the implementers to be involved in the planning, either directly or through representation. One need not be an expert to participate in the planning process. It is not necessary to know how to run a hospital or a unit to be involved in its planning. Any person who works in a hospital or uses one may contribute useful ideas about what services to provide and how to provide them. Effective organizational planning aims at satisfying its stakeholders, principally the customers and workers. The best way of doing this is to get them involved in designing the services in the first place. In the event you are wondering, I do mean involve the users (AKA patients) in the planning process.

Getting involvement from different workers and stakeholders of an organization in the planning process is usually easy; most workers want to be involved. A simple structure for doing so is to include people on the planning body from one or two administrative levels above and below the level that is being planned for (Ackoff, 1981). A diagram of this structure is in Figure 1.3.

Continuous Planning. Planning never ends. It is the ongoing work of the manager. It is *continuous*. To suggest otherwise is to deny the value of new information and to imply that you believe your planning assumptions are always correct. Plans once agreed on are never perfect and are rarely implemented as expected. Implementation has to be monitored, discrepancies

Figure 1.3. A Structure to Involve People in Planning.

EXTERNAL STAKEHOLDERS

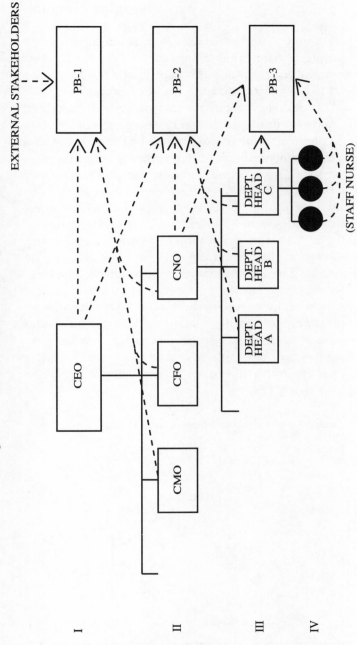

(STAFF NURSE)

Note: The roman numerals indicate organizational levels. Level I is the chief executive officer (CEO); Level II, the chief nursing officer (CNO) and counterparts for finance (CFO), medical staff (CMO), and so on; Level III, the nursing department or unit heads; and Level IV, staff nurses. PB indicates the planning body for the given level. For example, the planning body for the CNO (PB-2) would include the nursing department heads—and the CEO as well as the CNO. Others, for example, patients, the CMO, or external stakeholders, could be added as desired. The planning body for department head C (PB-3) includes all the staff nurses in the unit, or, if there are too many, some representative proportion; the CNO; and the head of nursing department C. This structure at the very least brings a manager into interactive contact with managers from one or two levels above and one or two levels below the level he or she occupies. Source: Adapted from Ackoff, 1981, p. 67.

between expected and actual outcomes noted, and feedback given to the appropriate decision maker for corrective action. Planning is not a once-a-year exercise; it is continuous. Or, as James Brian Quinn (1978) writes, planning is "evergreen."

"If it ain't broke, don't fix it" is a truism generally accepted by managers and popularly attributed to Bert Lance, President Jimmy Carter's first director of the Office of Management and Budget. Whether he actually was the originator is immaterial, because it is wrong! This sentiment not only impedes creativity in existing services, it accelerates their deterioration.

Actually, the time to "fix" something is before it breaks. Let me explain. Products and services have life cycles; the good ones go through phases of development, growth, and maintenance (plateau) and then generally decline, although they do not necessarily end. The curve shown in Figure 1.4 tells the story better than words.

This is what happens unless there is an intervention — an attempt to prevent or stop the decline. According to Lance, you should not mess with the curve until it is in its descendancy. That is bad advice, for the simple reason that it is much harder and more expensive to lift the curve than to keep it up in the first place (see Figure 1.5).

Figure 1.4. Product and Service Life Cycle.

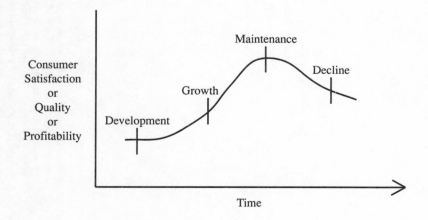

Figure 1.5. When It Is Not Broken *Is* the Time To Fix It.

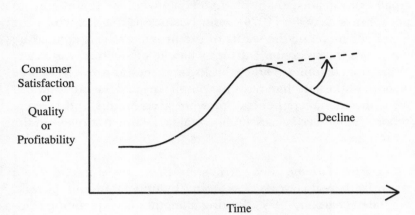

Note: The effort and expense needed to bring the life cycle curve back to growth or maintenance (arrow) are greater than capitalizing on momentum at the top of the curve. Keeping a service on top requires continuous planning and questioning of assumptions.

Of course, this means you have to examine the service before decline sets in, which means monitoring it over time as part of the planning process. You have to ask questions continuously about your services and management systems, even the best of them. Are they doing what was intended? Should they be changed? How can they be made better? Do they still fulfill our mission? What feedback are we getting from the stakeholders? This type of monitoring helps prevent decline because it does not allow us to take anything for granted. It forces us to question our assumptions, and unless we continuously question our assumptions about a service or a system, it will inevitably decline or fail.

Client Focus. Clients, customers, patients (the first two words are preferred because they have a service connotation, whereas the word *patients* does not) are to be served, and their well-being is ostensibly the reason hospitals exist. Of course, that is not the way it works. Hospitals are run more for the welfare and convenience of the people who work in them, principally physicians, than for the people who use them. But, to paraphrase Drucker (1974), your business is not defined by the hospital's name or the wants of the providers; it is defined by the wants the customer satisfies when he or she buys a service. What the customer wants, thinks, and sees at any given time is more important than what the physicians and the nurses want, what the managers believe, or what accountants and lawyers report. The more successful hospital is the one in tune with the customer.

Risk Taking. The purpose of planning is not to avoid risks. Rather, it is to *enable risk taking* by understanding the risks you take (Drucker, 1974). Putting it another way, planning helps you choose rationally among risk-taking courses of action. The increasing uncertainty in the health care world is a given, and the likelihood of greater uncertainty means greater risk. If risk is avoided, then change is avoided, and so too are the possibilities of developing and bettering your organization. Planning should prevent the uncritical extension of today's work into a risky tomorrow. (Tomorrow's risks are reduced if we do not assume that tomorrow's services, markets, and technologies will be the same as today's.)

Abandonment. Abandonment is a term Drucker (1974) uses to make the point that systematic abandonment of the old is just as important as systematic planning of the new and different. Hospitals are horrible at eliminating services and efforts that no longer satisfy the customer, fit the hospital's mission, or just do not work. Many full-service hospitals should not be full-service hospitals. By trying to do too much or more than resources allow to be done well, services suffer and patients become dissatisfied. Planning includes asking whether the hospital's existing services fit the realities of its population base, markets, technology, and available supporting resources.

Most of the hospital managers I know complain of being too busy, yet they continually add new tasks to their workload without ridding themselves of others. This means either that they are not really too busy or that they do not do a lot of what they do very well. (There are limits to the amount that can be done well, by anybody.) A fundamental question of the planning process is "If we weren't already doing _____ [you fill in the blank], would we begin to do it today?" Hospitals might consider, as a general rule, providing a new service or expanding an old one only while simultaneously eliminating or reducing an ongoing one. A criterion for doing something new ought to be whether or not you are willing to give up something to do it.

Creativity. When planning works, it unleashes our natural but suppressed creativity. Despite an educational system that rewards conformity more than uniqueness and the bureaucratic way of managing organizations with its practiced way of rejecting innovative ideas, creativity and innovative capacity lie in all of us, albeit dormant. Anyone observing children can tell you that they are highly creative, particularly at play or when not paying attention to adults. Children are creative because they do not think about constraints; they only think about what they want.

Creativity ends at school age, not because it is genetically programmed to last only five or six years, but because it is suppressed by adults who mistakenly equate it with lack of discipline. The different ideas of schoolchildren or employees often are stifled or ignored because they do not conform to existing ways of thinking or doing things, either in schools or in organizations. The school system aside, here are several suggestions for ways in which creativity can be activated in organizations through the planning process:

1. Reduce the exaggerated concern with facts and data collection that plagues typical planning and increase the organization's concern for ideas — all ideas. Obviously, a certain amount of information and data is necessary in planning. But the point here is that analytical overkill seldom is worth the effort, and it distracts you from what you should be about, namely, thinking creatively about what you want to do and be.

2. Suspend your concern for implementation until you decide what you want to do. Frequently, ideas are pursued on the basis of how they can or cannot be implemented. Rather, develop the ideas, add to them, change them, and play with them. Good ideas breed good ideas. Bringing implementation into your thinking too soon forecloses further thought and often leads to reasons for not doing something.

3. Recognize the inertia of habit. Fight against the reluctance to try something new simply because it has not been done before. Instead of looking for reasons why something will not work — for example, having nurses be responsible for patient management rather than physicians — ask yourselves how it can be made to work. Not all new or different ideas are worthy of trial, but you cannot find out the worth of an idea by rejecting it because it is different; it needs to be explored first.

4. Increase participation in the planning process. I have already emphasized participation, but I want to reemphasize it because it is directly related to creativity. Simply put, more creative ideas come from groups of people than individuals. Planning at the top of an organization limits the number of creative ideas to that particular handful of people. Treating everybody in the organization as planners increases the number of creative ideas.

5. Focus on why. Asking why something works or does not work leads to understanding. And understanding leads to creativity. It is particularly important to ask the "why" questions before the "how" questions.

Russell Ackoff (1981) uses a question to stimulate the release of creative thought in planning. To paraphrase it: If your hospital (or unit) were destroyed last night, what would you replace it with now — in its current environment? Asking this question releases you from the burden of defending the status quo and justifying current behavior, practices, assumptions, and goals. It enables you to start from scratch — and starting from scratch as a way of thinking is more creative because it enlarges your perspective of what is possible.

The beauty of this question is its simplicity. It removes the constraints (self-imposed) on our thinking by the obsession with problem solving and remediation that plagues managers. Asking "What would you replace your organization with if it were destroyed last night?" enables you to think as a child, without these constraints, because you focus on what you want, not what you do not want.

Steps in Planning

When the planning process works, the steps blend into one another. The order is not prescribed; it is fluid. The sequence can be started or entered at any point. A typical sequence is as follows:

1. Identifying and getting consensus around the values of the people planning for the organization. Determining what you want the organization to stand for, what you want it to be. The embodiment of this effort is the mission statement.
2. Determining what will happen if the organization does not change, if it continues the course it is on. This process helps you identify the differences (gaps) between what your organization is and what you want it to be.
3. Environmental analysis. Gathering just enough information about your environments (external and internal) to get you started, but not so much as to stall you.
4. Implementation planning. Making an action plan to help you narrow the gaps and get you closer to where you want to be.
5. Measurement and control. Initially implementing the action plan. Determining progress and outcome, learning, and changing the plan because of what you learn.

Mission Statements. The process of building consensus around the shared values that give rise to the goals of an organization is what creating or re-creating a mission statement is all about. The process means involving people throughout the organization, not just those at the top. The best-sounding mission statement is not very useful, or even taken seriously, unless those expected to carry it out, the implementers, have a hand in developing it.

Mission statements serve two functions. First, they are expressions of the shared values of an organization, or, to be more precise, of the shared values of the people who make an organization work. (An organization does not have inherent values; it takes on the values of the people who run it.) And if the organization wants to do well, its values match as closely as possible those of its customers. Mission statements reflect ideals. What do the organization's people want it to be? What is their vision?

Second, mission statements are enabling documents. They are guidelines for decision makers. This means they include more than general statements of philosophy and values; they indicate how the organization's values are to be applied. Here is an example of a hospital mission statement:

> The mission of _____ hospital is to provide comprehensive, high-quality health care and related services, in a sensitive and humane manner, to all who seek care. At all times the comfort and well-being of patients shall be of primary concern. Included in the mission is a dedication to the people who work in this hospital. The hospital intends to maintain an environment conducive to the continuing development of its employees. It recognizes that in today's environment the cost of health care services is a major factor in making health care decisions, and the hospital is concerned that the services it provides be economical as well as effective. Another aspect of its mission is to provide educational programs and clinical opportunities for the nurses and physicians to advance their knowledge so as to serve others in the future.

This is a typical mission statement. Many of you, perhaps too many, recognize it as one that approximates your own. Actually, it is a paraphrase of a mission statement of a large teaching hospital. Unfortunately, it is not complete; it is merely a statement of philosophy.

Statements of philosophy are not mission statements. By themselves, without elaboration, they are only platitudinous obeisance to motherhood and apple pie. We feel good and get warm, fuzzy feelings reading them, but they offer nothing useful to the various decision makers in your hospital or unit.

Take a closer look at the mission statement. What does *comprehensive* mean? What does *high-quality* mean? Are you really going to serve everyone who comes to your door? What are *related services* — are you going to operate a beauty salon or barbershop, or do you mean community education programs or a day-care center for disabled people? What does maintaining an environment conducive to the development of your employees mean in terms of tangible or measurable benefits? What types of training will be offered to nurses and physicians?

The mission statement example outlines several important goals, highly desired but meaningless unless turned into something more specific and measurable. (At least progress toward achieving goals should be measurable.) Goals have to be turned into specific objectives to help make good on the promises of your goals.

Now, we look at four excerpts from a twelve-page mission statement that are much more helpful to the managers of that hospital. Each is taken almost verbatim from the mission statement.

1. Service Mix — Centers of Excellence:

"While _____ cannot realistically be the best in everything it does, selected Centers of Excellence shall be emphasized. Rehabilitation, Burn Therapy, Occupational Medicine, Cardiology, Renal Disease, Fitness and Health Promotion, a Women's Center, and Geriatrics are all good candidates for special attention at this time. Others will be considered as opportunities arise."

2. Size — Growth:

"_____ shall grow through vertical integration of less costly external services such as Home Care, Outpatient

Surgery, Occupational Medicine, Fitness and Health Promotion, and Geriatrics by the geographic dispersion of both acute and ambulatory services.

"Growth for growth's sake will not be encouraged. Instead, _____ shall seek to grow by becoming better rather than bigger. Organizational units shall not expand to a size that precludes their ability to respond readily to changing market conditions.

"Depending on population growth and movement, the existing facility at _____ Street may be reduced in bed capacity during the next few years. Sites for possible satellite facility development shall be acquired in easily accessible areas of existing or potential population growth.

"In supporting this transformation, _____ shall be conservative in its use of debt. Caution will be exercised not to threaten long-term financial viability or short-term cashflow during this time of economic uncertainty."

3. Geographic Focus:

"For most of its programs and services, _____ will concentrate on the Greater _____ market. Some of its more regional programs, such as the Burn Center and Rehabilitative Medicine, will reach past this locale, but they will not compete with similar programs that have an obligation to serve their own regions. For example, burn patients from the _____ and _____ areas will not be sought. Special emphasis will be placed on discouraging indigent and government-reimbursed admission for less than billed charges from outside the _____ region of obligation.

"_____ will not seek to serve outlying areas in ways that tend to aggravate an already unacceptable uncompensated care situation."

4. Medical Education:

"The present and growing physician surplus in _____ and the advent of prospective pricing programs may have made graduate medical education program affiliation less desirable than it was under previous market conditions. Thus, _____ shall be more circumspect in its support of _____ Medical School and other similar programs. The direct pay-

ments and indirect expense of training the residents may place
_____ in a poor position, and each area of participation shall be studied to ensure that a strategic disadvantage is
not being created.

"_____ will maintain a limited affiliation with
the _____ Medical School to the extent that the relationship is beneficial to the community and serves the interests
of both institutions.

"The _____ primary mission of direct patient
care shall take precedence over the Medical School mission of
training new physicians and surgeons."

The first excerpt states that the hospital will not even attempt to be all things to all people. The areas of emphasis or
special attention are made explicit, and, at the same time, new
areas of concern as circumstances change are not precluded. The
decision maker, when asked to put more resources into another
service — for example, transplantation or obstetrics — has the im-
primatur to say no.

The second and third excerpts have to do with size and
growth. The service areas of growth are spelled out, growth for
its own sake is rejected, and a named facility is slated for reduction, pending specified evidence.

In the fourth excerpt, the issue of medical training is
raised. The prospect of curtailing such training is advanced,
but at the same time continuing medical education is declared
worthy of support. Significantly, the framers of this mission
statement identify the hospital's primary mission as patient
care; medical training is put into a subordinate position.

Although not complete objectives, these statements give
direction and guidance to the managers of the hospital. They
are enabling, that is, they allow managers to say yes or no to
requests for resources, new services, or modifications of existing ones. They enable marketing and purchasing decisions because they specify services and efforts within the hospital's mission and identify others to be excluded. And they identify for
its stakeholders what makes the hospital different from others.

Mission development is essential to the planning process.
Expressing values gives direction to the sorting-out process. It

helps us decide what to be, what to make of our environment, what opportunities to pursue, and what threats to repel. If sufficiently enabling and specific, a mission statement is instructional for the managers. A well-designed, operationally effective statement says to the decision maker: When you reach a point of critical choice, this is what you have to keep in mind.

But the goals of the mission statement have to be taken to the next step; they must be turned into measurable achievement—what I call objectives. This is the work of the people in the units and services. Their work flows from the values and guidelines of the mission statement that they helped devise and agreed on. (For examples of turning goals into objectives, see "Implementation Planning.")

Determining What Will Happen If the Organization Does Not Change. In 1990, the percentage of the GNP devoted to health care in the United States was approximately 11.5 percent. At the current rate of increase, it is estimated that by the year 2050, 100 percent of the GNP will be devoted to health care. Absurd? Yes! Ridiculous? Yes! But inaccurate? No! If nothing else changes or no interventions take place, 100 percent of the GNP will be devoted to health care in sixty years. The key words are *changes* and *interventions*. Something has to give. Some change or intervention or a series of them is certain because we know that all of our resources cannot be devoted to health care.

So, too, must some change or intervention take place to prevent harmful or excessive current practices and outcomes from causing irreparable damage later or placing our organizations in positions that require herculean efforts to change or use more resources than are available or we want to expend.

An example closer to home relates to the purported nursing shortage. Suppose your hospital has lost 5 percent of its nursing staff for each of the past three years. What happens if this decrease continues for three more years? Patient care suffers, the hospital cannot provide all the services it does now, more nurses leave because of the workload, and the hospital closes. All are possible outcomes.

Another example deals with expansion rather than contraction. Suppose that your intensive-care unit has thirty-six beds and has grown approximately 25 percent each of the past two years — that is, from twenty-four to thirty-six beds — and the unit no longer fits comfortably into the existing allocated space. If this growth continues, or, more accurately, if you allow it to grow at this rate without change, carrying the argument to the extreme, you will eventually have an intensive-care hospital and nothing else.

Typical responses to this situation are "How can we get more resources?" or "From what unit or activity should we divert resources?" A much better first series of questions is "Should the ICU continue to expand?" or "Do we need an ICU at all?" or "Does the ICU expansion fit into our mission?" or "Is expanding the ICU important enough to give up something else?"

It is essential to the planning process to ask continuously, "What happens if we continue our current way of doing things?" Ackoff (1981) calls the answers to these questions *reference projections*. The process entails projecting your organization to continue as it is without alterations, in either the organization or its external environment.

The assumptions underlying these projections are obviously false; your organization and its external environment will change. But thinking this way enables you to

1. Understand how the organization or unit might deteriorate if it continues as is
2. Identify what changes ought to be made (that is, make the right changes)
3. Identify some of the impediments to making the changes

Making reference projections is not forecasting. It is asking yourself "What happens if we don't change?" It is a determination of the future you are in if the organization continues as it is.

Environmental Analysis. If you wait for complete information before you implement, an opportunity may pass you by; it may be too late. Actually, if you have the time for complete analysis (if there is such a thing), the decision is not very important. See Figure 1.6.

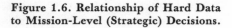

Figure 1.6. Relationship of Hard Data to Mission-Level (Strategic) Decisions.

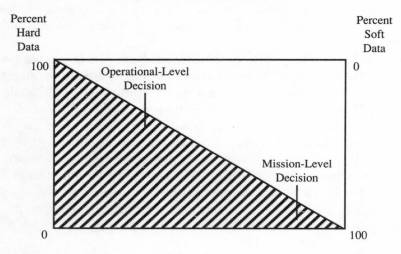

The mission-level decision is the one that may change your organization or improve its possibilities, the decision that may take the organization or a substantial part of it in a different direction. This is what some call a *strategic decision.* Examples are starting a new service or expanding an old one, redesigning your management system, eliminating a unit, changing emphasis, or cooperating with a competitor, in other words, anything that affects your mission, either to expand it or to cause you to think about changing it.

The operational-level decision is the decision about the way things are done — the who, how, when, and where. These decisions depend on having enough detailed knowledge, for example, to select personnel, beds, and equipment needed for a rehabilitation unit, identify the location for a satellite wellness clinic, choose between two different imaging devices, or equip a surgical suite.

The mission-level decision is generally made with less-than-complete information, often with relatively few hard data, and thus entails uncertainty. And uncertainty means risk. But if everything were certain, you would not have to plan. You would need only to decide what you wanted and go to it, because the outcomes would be known. Thus, planning can be thought of as a way of managing uncertainty.

Being informed reduces uncertainty. Relevant hard data help reduce uncertainty and improve decisions. The purpose of gathering data is to get answers to questions that help you make decisions and achieve goals. The key is to ask the right questions. Most managers I know suffer from having too much information. Most management information systems give their users much more information than they need or can use. Managers need information systems that produce much less in amount and much more in relevance. But the systems themselves are not at fault; information systems do only what they are asked (programmed) to do. If they are asked pertinent questions they will respond in kind. If they are asked for the universe of data, they will give it to you.

Information gathering should not take the form of an expedition; it should be purposeful. Facts are not important by themselves, but only in relationship to something you want to do and especially to understand. Before collecting information, ask yourself what you want to know, why you are gathering the data. The question should determine what kind of data you need. Are you starting a new service, such as a geriatric clinic or a women's health service? Then from your external environment you want to find out what kind of market you have for the service, if you have to develop a new market, what the perceptions of potential customers are (you have to ask them), what kind of competition you have — who it is and what it does — and more important than anything else, what you have to do so that customers will want to use your service rather than another. From your internal environment you want to find out if there are enough resources in the form of people, knowledge, money, space, and technology; if not, you need to learn what has to be done to get them.

Answering these types of questions does not require ex-

haustive data. Initial implementation needs only basic information, not encyclopedic knowledge. All that is required is enough
information to enable you to begin (or not to). Then you can
learn what additional information is needed as you go.

Examples of types of useful information are shown in the
following list. However, these are only illustrative. The depth
to which you pursue any of them should be related to obtaining
the minimum amount of information needed to take action, to
achieve an objective.

1. Stakeholders
2. Demographics
    • age shifts
    • catchment-area migration
3. Government
    • legislation
    • court decisions
4. Consumer attitudes and perceptions
    • wellness
    • education
    • convenience
5. Industry (employers)
6. Manpower
    • supply and distribution
    • trends in health practices
7. Competition
    • other hospitals
    • alternative delivery systems
    • physician groups
    • nursing facilities
8. Economic conditions
9. Medical technology
10. Changing values

The categories listed below represent the gamut that can be
run in gathering data. They range from people-based guesses to
sophisticated, computer-based simulation models, the latter, generally speaking, being less rewarding but more time consuming.

1. People-based:
   - guess
   - brainstorming
   - opinion consensus (Delphi)
2. Data-based:
   - data analysis
       trend extrapolation
       surveys
   - models
       simulation
3. Information sources:
   - publications
   - government statistics
   - conferences
   - individuals
       people served
       employees
       board members

   The people in your organization are a tremendous source of information. A manager or technician who has a friend working in another hospital can be the repository of a lot of information about a new management system or technology being used there or elsewhere. But this source has to be tapped, and the way to do this is to involve people in your planning. This is another reason why participation is so important to the planning process.

   Implementation Planning. Implementation is not a separate act; it is an integral part of planning. But implementation thinking is enhanced when it comes after you decide what your goals are — what you want — because, as I discussed under "Creativity," premature consideration of implementation inhibits creativity by foreclosing a full identification of alternatives. An unfettered exploration of the possibilities for your organization "after it was destroyed" leads to more creative ideas about goals and frequently results in imaginative implementation ideas. For example, when we initially planned the Johnson & Johnson-

Wharton Fellows Program, our principal goal was not to develop a high-quality management education program. Had this been the main goal, our implementation thinking most likely would have focused on topics and content, the usual considerations of educational programming. Instead, our goal was to design a program that would actually enable the participants to apply at least some of what was learned when they returned to their hospitals. This goal was more creative because it was what we really wanted, something seldom achieved in short-term education — people using what they learn.

Because of the way our goal was couched, we thought about implementation in terms of what to do to increase the likelihood of the educational content actually being used. So we asked ourselves what circumstances help people employ what they learn. One answer did not take long in coming: There is a much greater chance of using something you learned if at least one other person from your organization is with you, listening to the same words and learning at the same time. This thinking led to the design principle of the CEOs coming to the last two days of the program to work with the nurse executives on implementation issues.

Setting goals creatively, without the usual self-imposed constraints, without cries of "it won't work," "the boss won't like it," "it hasn't been done before," and "that's not the way we do things," leads to creative ideas about implementation as well. Implementation planning, then, is an extension of the creative effort of developing goals. Just as the mission statement is the embodiment of goal setting, a written action plan is the incarnation of implementation planning.

The components of an action plan are outlined below, and a description of each follows.

1. What you want to do
    *   objectives
    *   outcomes
2. Why you want to do it (the rationale)
    *   information from environments

- assumptions
3. Stakeholders
    - who has to be involved or informed
    - responsibility
4. Steps to be taken (the nitty-gritty)
    - what, when, where, how
5. Resources needed
    - people
    - money
    - information
    - facilities
    - technology
    - time
6. Measurement and control

I want to underscore the importance of putting action plans in writing. Organizations are not what the organizational charts suggest: nice, neat, well-defined linkages with clear distinctions about who does what, when, where, and how. They are, instead, loosely knit confederations of individuals following dotted-line relationships, ad hoc alliances, and even their own whims. This is the reason for a written action plan — some piece of writing that contains for all the protagonists to see (1) what is to be done; (2) why; (3) the names of who does what, when, where, and with what resources; and (4) no less important, how its accomplishment is to be gauged or measured.

The first step is *what you want to do*. This step requires you to think through what you want to do and to identify the criteria or specifications or outcomes that measure its achievement. This is the process of converting your goals (ideals) into specific objectives. In effect, you ask what you would take as evidence that your goal was achieved or how you would recognize its achievement (Mager, 1972).

For example, one of your goals may be "to have department heads manage their units effectively." This is a marvelous goal, but unless it is turned into something more concrete, an outcome that can be measured, it is essentially worthless. What does managing effectively mean? Let me relate what one group I worked with identified as the criteria and outcomes of effective department head management. The six criteria were:

1. Less than 5 percent absenteeism on the unit
2. Staff turnover less than 10 percent
3. Does not exceed budget
4. Less than 10 percent of patients with complaints
5. Recruits fifteen nurses within six months
6. Shows responsibility

After further deliberation, this group discarded the sixth criterion ("shows responsibility") because it was too vague. While not exhaustive or pertinent to every department, the remaining five criteria are valid measures. They can be used to determine whether a department is managed effectively. You can add others or change these as your own circumstances warrant. But without specific criteria the goal remains abstract and unmeasurable. Stating the criteria changes the goal to a measurable objective.

Another, more global example again shows the value of thinking through what you want and what you would accept as evidence that your goal was achieved. Quality is certainly a concern for all hospitals. Measuring quality, according to many people who provide medical and health care, is difficult or impossible. Is it? I worked with a physician who was responsible for a rehabilitation unit, and her goal was "to provide high-quality care to people in the rehabilitation unit of _____ hospital." What follows are the criteria she decided, after some thought, would be reasonable measures of such a unit.

1. Average length of stay equal to or less than the average for the diagnostic classification
2. Restoration to function (complete self-care) according to disability classification exceeds average within the time span of twelve weeks
3. Frequency of changing initial treatment goals less than 15 percent

4. Less than 10 percent avoidable medical complications such as or including:
   - decubitus ulcers
   - medication errors
   - patient falling out of bed because side rails not raised, and so forth
5. Provision of a nursing care plan for family or nursing home: for example, follow-up appointments for speech therapy, physical therapy, and so on; maintenance and repair instruction
6. Greater than 80 percent positive responses from patients to a questionnaire concerning their care
7. Greater than 80 percent positive responses from family to a questionnaire concerning:
   - follow-up care
   - their understanding of problem

These criteria are not necessarily the last word, but they are reasonable measures of high-quality rehabilitative care. A unit achieving at this level is a good one by anybody's standards.

The same process can be applied to virtually any goal, clinical or managerial. Remember, most goals are abstract expressions of something important to you, your values, your ideals (Mager, 1972). For example, you have a physical examination to determine your health, but nobody checks your health, because health is an abstraction. It is the specifics — for example, your blood pressure, pulse rate, temperature, blood chemistry, and mental outlook — that collectively measure your health, that turn the abstract into the concrete. The same holds for your organization and its goals (mission). How do you measure the "health" of your hospital? Do the customers (patients) get appropriate high-quality care with few errors and inconveniences? Do they prefer your services to those of other hospitals? Do the people who work in the hospital like working there? Do they feel they participate in goal setting? Do they know what is going on? Is the hospital sound fiscally? Are the vicissitudes of the external environment confounding, or are responses made less than hysterically? Is planning an ongoing function? Is monitoring performance threatening or looked upon as a learning mechanism? The answers to these and related questions are the specifics that measure the "health" of your hospital. Goals (what your organization wants to be) have to be turned into objectives — what you want to do so that you can be what you want to be.

Next is the question of *why you want to do it (the rationale)*. It is my observation that many objectives are pursued and efforts undertaken without really identifying or understanding why. For example, your hospital is urged by either external or internal stakeholders to open an addiction treatment unit. The reasons given are that other hospitals have such units, and drug problems are a major societal problem. And your decision makers assume it is a good thing to do.

But is it good for you to do it? There are questions to ask before acting on this assumption. For instance, how will this unit improve your hospital? How many will benefit? Why will addicts come to your service rather than another? What impact will it have on existing services? Does it fit the mission, and, if not, is it important enough to change the mission? Are the resources needed better applied in support of another, more broadly desired service? What happens if you do not do it?

Thoroughly assessing why you want to do something and the validity of your supporting assumptions helps separate what is good to do (which is limitless) from what is best to do in terms of providing a superior service to your customers. It leads to sounder decisions and also links planning assumptions with outcomes, which makes diagnosis and revision easier when implementation outcomes fail to match expectations.

Planning assumptions should be carefully probed not only when goals are set but on an ongoing basis as well. Many organizations spend a lot of energy and resources doing the wrong things, efficiently. Running a highly efficient neonatology service matters little when it has a low utilization rate due to a large decrease in couples of child-bearing age in your community.

A useful way to avoid doing the wrong things, efficiently or not, is to keep reminding yourself why you are doing something. This means reexamining the assumptions behind your decisions. We tend to do things because we are used to doing them, and it is comfortable to keep doing them, even though the original assumptions and reasons that prompted the effort no longer apply. Writing down the assumptions, reasons, and data that give rise to expanding a service, adding a unit, or changing a system, for example, enables the decision makers to validate the grounding for these actions as a routine part of planning and when problems crop up.

The *stakeholders* represent a third consideration. Implementation means that people do things. Responsibility is given and taken. When implementation does not work well, a significant factor has to do with how well and how clearly responsibility is given and accepted. Frequently, people, sometimes in large numbers, believe that responsibility resides in one place when, in fact, it is lodged somewhere else. Who is responsible for what and how one individual's responsibility is perceived by another or oneself are real issues in implementation. These matters are discussed in depth in Chapter Nine. A related issue, negotiation, is considered in Chapter Ten. Many managers consider this part of planning tedious, as interesting as watching paint dry, and unworthy of consuming time that could better be spent on "more important" efforts. As a result, details are frequently neglected and implementation suffers. Many an innovation or good idea goes down the drain and is mistakenly judged to be not such a good idea after all because the specifics of implementation are given inadequate attention. But the quality of thought given to *who does what, when, where, and how* is the chief determinant of whether something will work.

It does not take a lot of time, but it does take some time to think through these details. And it does not have to be done to the *nth* degree, in final form. It only has to be done to the extent that it enables the effort to begin and those responsible for its outcomes to learn what modifications are needed.

The *resources needed* also have to be evaluated. There are two considerations for resource planning: the types of resources, and an estimate of how much of each resource is needed. The types of resources are people, money, information, facilities, technology, and—one that is often overlooked—time. Time is usually given short shrift in the calculus of resource planning. Of all the resources time is the most underestimated. It seems to be a human idiosyncrasy that we believe a task can be accomplished in less time than it actually takes, particularly if we have not done it before. One guess is that it is much easier to say than to do. Another reason is that we do not think things through well enough to account for the myriad details that consume time. And we cannot foresee all the problems that inevitably occur. Implementation means detail and foul-up, and both mean time.

Measurement and Control. But it really is not possible to think through every detail of achieving an objective or completing a project beforehand; you have to get into it. You have to get into it to find out what works, what does not work, and why. Real accuracy about resource requirements comes after the effort is under way, not before. This means that the initial allocation of resources and decisions about how much money is needed, the number and types of personnel, the information required, and the necessary space and technology are made in terms of what you think it takes to get something started and going to the extent that you can learn from it.

Measurement and control represent the learning-feedback-modification stage. They involve adapting and revising your effort and the further deployment of supporting resources if necessary because of what you learn by measuring the discrepancies between actual and expected performance or outcomes, and especially because of what you learn about what caused them.

A plan represents only what the planners thought important and wanted at the time it was conceived. The future seldom conforms to expectations; outcomes seldom reflect exact intentions; assumptions prove false; and conditions (environments) change between the time a plan is prepared and its implementation. So revision and change are necessary. They are as much a part of the planning process as is goal setting. Frequent revision is not indicative of poor planning (Peters, 1979). Just the opposite. Revision means you keep track of what you do, think about it, make necessary changes, and do not regard what is done as immutable.

Deciding what you want may be more fun, but measuring and revising what you do, although more difficult and painful (it is not pleasant to identify efforts gone wrong and mistaken assumptions), are more closely connected to achievement. But the question is, what do you measure? My answer is that you measure whether you are getting what you want — that is, the progress toward and achievement of your goals and objectives — and if you are not achieving them, why not. Yet managers concentrate their measurement efforts on something else, namely, what is readily quantifiable and easiest to measure: occupancy rates, number of procedures, revenues, expenses, space used, depreciation, and the like. While these data should be known, they are less important than knowing, for example, whether the services your hospital or unit provides are appropriate, what the people who use your services think about them, and why you fail to attract both employees to work in your hospital and people to use your services.

Significant discrepancies between desired outcomes and actual performance should be detected as quickly as possible so that corrections and revisions can be made before the discrepancies become crises. Constant monitoring and feedback are essential. This means, of course, that responsibility for monitoring is assigned and accepted and made known.

When discrepancies are noted, think first about your assumptions. Are they valid? Do they still fit your environmental analysis? Has the environment (external or internal) changed enough to warrant different assumptions? For example, demographic shifts resulting in different service markets, more prevention- and health-conscious consumers requiring more education and less intervention, and significant changes in staffing or unavailability of certain personnel needed for technological complexity should cause a reexamination of the assumptions that guide your service mix.

If your assumptions are valid and the objective is sound, then check the implementation for the cause of the discrepancy. Was the service marketed adequately? Did you give the effort enough time? Do the personnel match the requirements? Is responsibility clear? Are there internal obstructions in the form of bruised egos or individual recalcitrance?

After all this, you may conclude that the goal is inappropriate or unachievable for lack of resources. In the first instance, consider abandoning it, and in the second, think about integrating the program or service with another, or diverting resources from elsewhere; but keep in mind the hazards to the existing programs of doing so.

The "why" concerns that lead to understanding, although always difficult to measure, are the most important because they tell you more about your hospital and its practices than the quantifiable data mentioned. Getting what you want, achieving your goals, is advanced more by knowing (measuring) why something works or does not work than by being familiar with the numbers on computer printouts. As Ackoff (1986) writes, it is better to measure imprecisely what is wanted than precisely what is not.

A Planning Design

Instead of a summary, I leave you with a planning design that brings together the parts of the process into a coherent whole (see Figure 1.7). The design may seem peculiar, particularly if you are habituated to the linear planning models with their boxes, lines, and arrows illustrated earlier in Figures 1.1 and 1.2. But the overlapping, amoebalike configuration portrays the fluid, ever-changing, continuous concept of planning that I want to advance. External and internal environments change as does your organization's mission. Together they shape a working plan — what you want to do — that is not fixed; the plan changes as you learn from implementation what needs changing. No matter how many data you collect, how long you plan, and how orderly and manageable it looks on paper, you do not know if your plan — for example, a new service or a change in an existing one — will work or will be profitable until you try it. So the planning design is not whole until implementation, the learning ingredient, is included.

Trying something, experimentation, is a precursor to learning. Hard data lead to learning, and the quickest route to

Figure 1.7. A Planning Design.

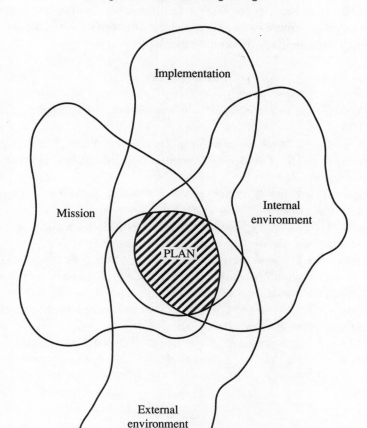

hard data is experimentation. There are no solutions with respect to the future; there are only alternative courses of action, each imperfect, each risky, each uncertain, each requiring different efforts and costs (Drucker, 1974). The manager's job is to choose among them. But the alternative that works cannot be known until it is put into action — tried.

This planning design is built around constant constructive

38 Managing Hospitals

change and depends on results, especially what is learned from implementation. Its success or failure depends on what you do, not what is done to you. If, then, the future is a moving target, this design helps you take better aim.

References

Ackoff, R. L. *Creating the Corporate Future*. New York: Wiley, 1981.
Ackoff, R. L. *Management in Small Doses*. New York: Wiley, 1986.
Drucker, P. F. *The Age of Discontinuity*. New York: Harper & Row, 1969.
Drucker, P. F. *Tasks, Responsibilities, Practices*. New York: Harper & Row, 1974.
Hurst, D. K. "Why Strategic Management Is Bankrupt." *Organizational Dynamics*, 1986, *15* (2), 5–27.
Mager, R. F. *Goal Analysis*. Belmont, Calif.: Fearon, 1972.
Peters, J. P. *Strategic Planning for Hospitals*. Chicago: American Hospital Association, 1979.
Quinn, J. B. "Strategic Change: Logical Incrementalism." *Sloan Management Review*, 1978, *19*, 7–21.
Toffler, A. *Future Shock*. New York: Bantam, 1971.

CHAPTER 2

Utilizing Marketing
in the Planning Process

Elizabeth F. Dunn

In the past few years, hospital managers at all levels have become accustomed to the idea of having a marketing department in the hospital. Managers understand that reduced admissions, increasing competition, and shaky financial situations have made marketing a necessity. But many managers still feel some level of discomfort about the idea of marketing health services. In seminars on health care marketing, when health care managers are asked to "say whatever comes into your minds when you hear the word *marketing*," managers first cite various marketing functions such as "advertising" and "selling." Then, as they continue to free-associate, they inevitably produce more evaluative phrases like "manipulating people" and "getting people to buy what they don't really need." And one or more managers usually say, "I know that our hospital has to do marketing, if only because all of our competitors do it, but I'm still not totally comfortable with it. It doesn't seem to 'go' with health care."

This discomfort with marketing reflects lingering confusion as to what marketing really is. Marketing can be defined as follows: (1) finding out what the customer wants/needs, and (2) fulfilling those needs better than anyone else while (3) meeting your financial objectives. When viewed in this way, it is obvious that marketing is not a new concept for hospitals. It has actually been practiced in hospitals for hundreds of years. Clinicians and administrators have always attempted, with varying degrees of success, to determine what patients need and to fill those needs. What is new in the past ten years is that the tools of modern marketing have been applied to the hospital setting in a systematic and sophisticated way. What is also new is the realization that determining what consumers want and need is so important to institutional strength and survival that it needs the attention of a *full-time* and *specialist* staff. And finally, in this new competitive and cost-conscious environment, marketing performs another "new" function. Since not all health care services can be provided profitably, marketing can help prevent unrealistic expectations on the part of the hospital and its doctors by analyzing the market potential and true marketing costs of services being planned.

A Review of the Basics

Two key marketing concepts are described below. These, along with the 4 P's of marketing (to be discussed in the next section), constitute the repertoire of knowledge managers require to understand the issues of marketing.

Target Marketing. To fulfill their service-oriented missions, most hospitals have traditionally attempted to provide services to everyone who wanted them. In recent years, however, hospitals have designed and communicated services for specific *target markets*. Some examples of targeted services follow:

- Fitness services for twenty-five- to forty-five-year-old healthy adults
- Senior citizen clubs for people sixty-five and over
- "Gold Coast" inpatient facilities for the affluent
- Women's centers for women aged eighteen to sixty-five

It is important to note that specifying a target market is not designed to exclude those not in the target market. For example, few hospitals would deny access to their seniors' club to a forty-five-year-old who wished to join. Rather, the objective of defining a target market is to enable the marketer to accomplish two objectives: (1) to research that one particular target market in depth so that its characteristics, needs, and desires can be learned, and (2) to develop a clear, concrete image of one specific group of customers when she or he is designing the product or service, the physical location, the pricing, and the promotional materials for the product or service.

There are many possible bases for selecting target markets, such as *gender* (the women's center) and *age* (senior center). These types of bases provide grounds for *demographic segmentation*. (*Segmentation* refers to dividing the entire market into submarkets on the basis of one or more variables.) Target markets can also be selected on the basis of *psychographic segmentation,* whereby the market is divided along psychological characteristics, usually on the basis of an extensive research study of the market.

An example of psychographic segmentation is a study of 2,000 consumers by Peabody Marketing Decisions, a San Francisco consulting firm. Peabody asked these consumers about their attitude on choosing health care services and, through statistical analysis, found that consumers fell into distinct psychographic categories or segments, including: the "quality minded," who are willing to pay extra for high-quality services; the "naturalists," who try alternative methods of health care services; the "health care avoiders," who only use emergency services; the "generics," who buy health care services on the basis of price alone; and the "loyalists," who have faith in providers.

Once a target market has been selected, it should be evaluated against the following criteria:

> *Size.* Is the target market large enough to sustain your program? If you are designing a daytime fitness program for nonworking mothers, are there enough nonworking mothers in your area to make it worthwhile?
> *Competitive Activities Directed at Your Target Segments.* Is your target market so attractive that it is already besieged by offers from other organizations? Is your group of nonworking mothers already being courted by compet-

itors' fitness or recreational programs? Remember, if a target segment is attractive to you, it is probably also attractive to competitors.

Reachability. Some target markets are theoretically attractive but difficult to reach from a communications standpoint. For example, you might decide to target a psychographic segment such as the health care avoiders. But it would be difficult to communicate effectively with a group who use only emergency services. Mass media would be inefficient and direct mail difficult.

Positioning. Once a target market has been selected and a product or service designed to meet its needs, the next step is to position the product. The object of positioning a product is to create a clear impression of your product in the customer's mind that fulfills two requirements: (1) the image should be based on one or two key product characteristics that are important to the customer, and (2) the image and the key characteristics should be different from those of your competitors. Companies have used many key characteristics as a basis of their positioning strategies. Typical characteristics include lowest price, highest quality, best service, and most reliability.

Once you select a basis for positioning, you need to incorporate it into every aspect of your marketing strategy. Consider a hospital that decides to use a "high-prestige" positioning strategy. That hospital needs to make sure that it does in fact have the highest-prestige physicians, staff, and environment in the area. Every communication that the hospital makes with its many audiences should include some indication of high-prestige positioning: advertising, public relations, stationery, even T-shirts.

Of course, positioning a hospital as high prestige is only meaningful if research has shown that potential customers view high prestige as an important attribute *and* if competitors are not using the same positioning. One hospital positioned itself as "the largest" in the area, only to learn that potential customers had some negative feelings about this attribute.

The 4 P's

By now, most hospital managers have some acquaintance with the "4 P's" of marketing: product, physical distribution, price, and promotion. But it may be helpful to review them.

Product. A product is most usefully described as a bundle of benefits as perceived by the customer. Thus, a kidney-stone lithotripter service is not "selling" the lithotripter. Instead, it is "selling" relief from discomfort, reduction of the risk that would have been incurred in surgery, and faster recovery relative to a surgical procedure. When designing or promoting a clinical service, it is extremely important to have a strong understanding of what the product — the bundle of benefits — is from the customer's perspective so that these benefits can be incorporated into the product and emphasized in promotional materials. In order to understand accurately what these benefits are, it is necessary to obtain the customer perspective by doing market research.

Failing to do homework (that is, market research) can result in costly errors. For example, some hospitals designed expensive fitness centers, based on the belief that consumers would find it to be a tremendous benefit that these centers were "medically supervised" and "affiliated with a hospital facility." Many of these hospitals learned the bitter lesson that these attributes were not perceived as significant benefits by consumers, and could in fact be perceived as liabilities.

Physical Distribution. In health care, the concept of physical distribution refers primarily to the site or location where clinical services are provided. Some examples of innovations in the physical distribution of services in recent years are as follows:

• The construction of freestanding surgicenters where an ever-increasing number of same-day surgical procedures are performed

- Vans that are converted into mobile diagnostic units and that go from neighborhood to neighborhood, providing a wide range of health-screening tests
- Designing breast-imaging centers for women that are separate from radiology services, attractively decorated, and accessible to outpatients at street level, instead of being located in the "bowels" of the hospital
- Location of an increasing number of diagnostic and therapeutic procedures in stylishly decorated physicians' offices, for example, lithotripsy and MRI
- An increasing number of substance abuse and other mental health services situated in locations throughout the community, designed to provide convenient and accessible services to the consumer

In general, the trend in health care is to provide services in locations that provide the maximum amount of convenience and accessibility to the consumer. For most health care services, consumers prefer locations that are close to home, in safe locations where their visitors can park without fear of crime, and convenient to public transportation. For some types of health services, such as substance abuse rehabilitation, consumers may prefer locations that are *not* close to home, so that their privacy is optimized.

The best rule of thumb for determining the optimal physical location for a service is to *ask the consumer*. Although the consumer's preference must always be put in the context of clinical and regulatory considerations, even the highest-quality clinical services will be underutilized if they are located at a site that does not fulfill consumer preferences.

The physical distribution of health care services is an area that holds enormous potential for creative innovation. Twenty years ago people would have been amazed to see the scope and sophistication of services that today are provided outside the four hospital walls. Twenty years or less into the future, we may be seeing diagnostic or even therapeutic services provided in the home via the patient's home computer.

Price. Of all the 4 P's — product, physical distribution, price, and promotion — the most complicated one in health care is price, for the following reasons. First, third-party payers put heavy constraints on the prices that health care providers can charge. Second, most consumers do not know the total price of a hospital procedure, whether it is an outpatient x-ray or a heart transplant, before they have it performed. Third, consumers vary widely in terms of the percentage of their hospital bill that they pay out of their own pocket. For a $5,000 hospital stay, one person's insurance will cover the entire amount, a second person will pay $1,000 out of pocket, and a third person will pay the entire $5,000 out of pocket. Fourth, health care is one of a variety of services and products that are subject to the *price-value paradox.* When the quality of a service or product is complex and difficult to evaluate, there is a tendency to believe that the more expensive product is the better product. For example, suppose that people are shown two luxury watches that are similar in appearance and brand reputation. One watch costs $300 and the other costs $230. If you ask these consumers which of the two watches is the better-quality watch, they will tend to say that the more expensive watch is the better one. The same is true in health care. Consumers often believe that because Hospital A is generally more expensive than Hospital B, Hospital A must be providing higher-quality care than Hospital B. Of course, in reality this may not be the case. Hospital A may be more expensive for a wide variety of reasons: It may have a heavy debt load from recent construction, or it may be inefficient in managing its cost. However, in marketing, it is the consumer's *perception* of price and quality that counts. Reality is secondary!

Because of these complexities in the way consumers view health care prices, few hospitals have taken the risk of using price as a marketing tool. Some examples follow.

In an effort to boost declining inpatient admissions, a number of hospitals have run advertisements that offer to accept Medicare as payment in full for inpatient stays. A possible disadvantage of this discounting strategy is based on the price-value paradox. Although some Medicare patients may be attracted to the hospital because of the discount, other consumers may perceive that the discounting is a reflection of poor quality and may be "turned off." The danger here is that managers can become distracted by the advantages of the discounting strategy (we increased admissions by 5 percent this month) and can be unaware of the erosion of the hospital's image that is occurring in the community.

A second example concerns the "package prices" that are provided for selected procedures. You may have seen newspaper ads that offer a "maternity package" for $1,500 or a cosmetic surgery package for $800. The maternity package might include prenatal and postnatal services from hospital staff physicians as well as all hospital charges. This maternity package price is usually slightly less than the standard price, and it is designed to increase admissions to an OB service that is underutilized. The "package" aspect of the price appeals to the consumer's lack of knowledge and confusion about all the various charges and costs involved in maternity and birthing care. Cosmetic surgery provides another illustration. The strategy of using a package price for this type of surgery has some unique advantages. Cosmetic surgery is one of the few clinical procedures that are rarely covered by health insurance. Since the consumer typically pays all the charges out of pocket, she or he is much more sensitive to the price than health care consumers usually are. Therefore, a price package or any type of price appeal is much more likely to succeed for plastic surgery than for other procedures. The concept of price packages is new in health care, and the final results are not yet in. In general, the advantage of attracting additional patients must be balanced against the erosion of the hospital's image due to "discounting."

It is clear, then, that the use of price as a marketing tool is very problematic in health care. A further complication in its use is that we cannot learn much from the economics and marketing literature in our attempt to understand the relationship between price and consumer behavior. The economics and marketing research simply does not apply to most health care situations, because that research does not address situations in which (1) the consumer often does not select the service (the doctor does); (2) some consumers pay a lot for the service and some pay nothing (depending on their insurance coverage); and (3) consumers often do not know the total price of a procedure until after it is performed. Only through pricing research specifically dedicated to the health care setting can we better understand the effectiveness of pricing as a marketing tool in health care.

Promotion. In health care, *promotion* refers to all the ways health care providers systematically communicate with their consumers to meet the organization's marketing objectives. In the "early days" of health care marketing, marketing and promotion were almost synonymous. For this reason, hospitals have had more experience with promotion than they have with other marketing mix variables. This extensive experience has led to a wide variety of promotional strategies, including the use of all print and electronic mass media (television, radio, magazine, newspaper, billboard, direct mail).

Initially, hospitals used advertising and other communications to portray their image. The problem with this approach was that most hospitals selected the same image to portray (that is, the "high-tech/high-touch" image). Overnight, hospitals from coast to coast began spending millions of dollars on television, magazine, newspaper, and billboard ads that looked very similar to one another. The basic recipe for these ads was a picture of one or more clinical staff members, usually standing next to either a patient or a piece of sophisticated machinery, and reassuring the audience that "At our hospital, we combine the highest level of clinical and technological expertise with the most caring attitude toward our patients."

The impact of this wave of "We Care" ads was negligible. Because most of the ads gave out the same message, consumers could not remember which hospital sponsored the ad. Also, most consumers do not select the hospital that they are going to for inpatient procedures. The decision is heavily influenced by physician recommendation.

New Advertising Strategies

For three or four years, millions of dollars of advertising money were spent on image ads with little or no impact. Recently, however, hospital marketers have begun to base their advertising strategies on two key factors: the hospital's strategic marketing objectives and the customer decision-making process.

Strategic Marketing Objectives. The strategic marketing objectives of a hospital should flow from the hospital's overall strategic plan. Some typical strategic marketing objectives are: increasing admissions by X percent; increasing profitability by X percent; increasing market share by X percent. A few things about these objectives are worth noting:

1. *Increasing admissions and increasing market share are very different objectives.* Let's say that in 1987 you had 20,000 admissions and there were a total of 80,000 admissions in your service area. Your market share would be 25 percent for the year. Then, in 1988, you had the same number of admissions — 20,000 — but the total number of admissions in your service area declined to 60,000. Your market share would be 33.33 percent. Thus, although you had the *same number of admissions* from 1987 to 1988, your *market share increased* dramatically because of a decline in the total market. Because hospital markets cannot influence the total number of admissions in the service area, hospitals prefer to use an increase in market share as a strategic objective, instead of an increase in admissions. If your annual admissions are declining but your market share is increasing (or even holding steady), your organization is doing a good job in marketing.

2. *"Increasing occupancy" is not a valid strategic marketing objective.* In the days of cost-based reimbursement, increased occupancy was generally viewed as a positive outcome. This was because, in most cases, the higher the occupancy, the greater the reimbursement revenue that the hospital received. Today this situation has changed dramatically. All Medicare patients and many privately insured patients are under prospective payment systems. Thus, exceeding DRG trim points can result in financial losses for the hospital. Even for those patients who are covered by some sort of cost-based reimbursement, increasing occupancy is not a valid marketing objective. Occupancy is determined by the number of admissions and the length of stay. Length of stay is determined by clinical events and physician judgment, neither of which is influenced by marketing efforts.

Focusing on strategic marketing objectives has led hospital marketers to alter their advertising strategies significantly. In the past, hospitals made decisions about placing their image advertisements based on the following motivation: to enhance the *image* of the hospital; to increase *awareness* of the hospital in the community; because other hospitals were doing it. Because there were no explicit strategic objectives underlying the advertising strategy, there was in most cases no way to measure objectively whether the ads were effective. Today hospitals are not only clearer about their strategic marketing objectives but also are more focused on measuring the effectiveness of advertising in helping to accomplish these objectives. Although evaluating the impact of advertising on marketing share or profitability is difficult in all industries, hospitals have made a start through a variety of approaches.

The Decision-Making Process. In addition to tying advertising strategies to strategic marketing objectives, hospital marketers have also begun to base their marketing (including advertising) strategies on a better understanding of the buyer *decision-making process.* This process is the single most important element of a marketing strategy. You can have a thorough understanding of your product, your price, and every aspect of advertising. But if you fail to understand the buyer decision-making process, you will not be able to focus your strategies effectively. The expenditure of millions of dollars by hospitals on image advertising in the early days of hospital marketing is a vivid example of this principle.

The buyer decision-making process consists of two elements: the decision-making unit and the decision-making process. These elements vary according to the product or service under consideration. Some examples are as follows:

Routine Purchase: Laundry Detergent

Decision-making unit	Primary grocery store shopper in household
Decision-making process	Shopper habitually purchases same brand. Some-

times this habit pattern is "disrupted" by a coupon or a discount.

Impulse Purchase: Earrings

Decision-making unit	Consumer
Decision-making process	Consumer walking down street, not intending to make purchase. Eye caught by gold earrings in window. Consumer calculates brief cost-benefit analysis, enters store, purchases earrings.

High-Involvement Purchase: Automobile

Decision-making unit	Consumer, spouse, older children, perhaps financial adviser
Decision-making process	Reading consumer product magazines, discussions with friends, many trips to dealers for comparison shopping, consensus among members of decision-making unit, purchase.

Health Care Service Selection: Inpatient Care

Decision-making unit	Patient, significant others, physician
Decision-making process	Patient selects physician, based on a number of criteria that may include physician's hospital affiliation. Physician specifies or recommends hospital, giving consumer varying degrees of choice. Usually consumer accepts physician recommen-

> dation. If not, consumer
> may select another physi-
> cian.

There are several key points to remember about decision-making processes. First, decision-making processes differ significantly depending on the type of product or service involved. Even within a hospital, decision-making processes are different for inpatient services, outpatient services, drug rehabilitation services, home health services, and emergency room services. And even within emergency room services, at least two types of decision-making processes have been identified: one for patients in emergency situations and one for patients who come to the ER for primary care treatment.

    Second, because decision-making processes are different for different services, they must be analyzed specifically for each service. Understanding the decision-making process for inpatient care does not help in understanding how ER patients select an emergency room. Even for obstetrics patients, the decision-making process differs somewhat from the one for surgical inpatient care. The key to the decision-making process lies with the consumer's psychology. It is always risky to assume that you, the manager, know what is in the consumer's mind. A true understanding of the consumer decision-making process can be gained only through market research, usually of the focus-group variety.

    Third, any marketing (including advertising) strategy should be based on the decision-making process. When hospital markets gained a better understanding of the consumer decision-making process, their marketing and advertising strategies for inpatient services changed. They changed or greatly reduced their newspaper and magazine ads to consumers and created new marketing strategies that acknowledged the influential role of the physician. Some examples of their strategies include: consumer advertisements that featured the hospital's leading physicians or groups of physicians; consumer advertisements that advertised the hospital's physician referral services; and ads that focused on services in which physician referral or influence was less important, such as obstetrics, ER services, and sports medicine programs.

Nurse Recruitment: A Marketing Application

Marketing tools are not limited to the standard problems of increasing market share or increasing profitability. Frequently, these tools may be applied to a variety of issues and problems facing the hospital.

One of the most serious issues facing hospitals today is the recruitment of nurses. Several hospitals have used marketing strategies to address this problem. An extended example involving the hypothetical "Alpha Hospital" follows.

Alpha Hospital began by setting two strategic objectives: (1) to increase the net number of staff nurses by twenty within one year, and (2) to have 80 percent of new hires remain on the staff for at least two years.

Alpha Hospital defined its target market as academically qualified nurses who had graduated from nursing school during the past academic year and who lived within a specified geographic radius of the hospital. Note that Alpha Hospital created a narrow target market for this strategy—that is, only recent graduates. This was a deliberate decision on Alpha's part and was based on its desire to gain an in-depth understanding of the segment. Alpha also attempted to recruit nurses from other hospitals but used a different strategy to do so.

In this strategy the decision-making process to be understood was "How do graduating nurses make a decision to select one hospital offer over another?" To understand this process, Alpha Hospital conducted focus groups among members of the target market. (See the section "Understanding the Customers' Needs," below, for a full description of focus groups.)

Two such groups were formed, each consisting of ten recent graduates from the area. All participants had interviewed for jobs, although not all had accepted them. The discussion was led by a marketing manager, who based his questions on a discussion guide. The discussion guide included questions on the decision-making process, perceptions of area hospitals, experiences during interviews, and reactions to recruitment ads.

It was created by a group consisting of a marketing manager, a human resources manager, and two nursing managers. The discussion was observed through a one-way mirror by interested managers.

Results of the focus group were summarized in written form and circulated among nursing and human resources managers. Based on the results, managers learned much about how recent graduates made the decision about which hospital to select. Because there are significant regional differences among recent graduates, the details will not be related here. However, some general findings are as follows:

- Students investigated an extremely large number of hospitals.
- Some investigations were very superficial and consisted of nothing more than telephone calls.
- Graduates were heavily influenced by opinions of their friends and would frequently rule out a hospital on that basis alone.
- Several graduates reported that they were personally uncomfortable with some of the people who interviewed them.
- Responses to recruitment ads were very informative. Some of Alpha Hospital's favorite ads were found to be "too cutesy" by participants.
- Participants wanted to be part of a stable environment, not one that was financially shaky. Participants felt that Alpha Hospital was much more financially stable than other area hospitals.

Alpha Hospital decided to position itself as "the stable, financially secure hospital in the area." Alpha selected this positioning partly because it was based on a dimension that was considered important to the target audience, and also because it was perceived to be different from its competitors along this dimension. Being stable and financially secure was not the most important factor in the decision process; highest salary was. But Alpha Hospital could not position itself as offering the highest salary because, in fact, it did not. Positioning is a matter of selecting the most important (to consumers) benefit that you *can* provide and that differentiates you from competitors.

As a result of the focus groups, management began to conceptualize the entire recruitment and interviewing process as part of the "product" they were offering. Before the focus groups, management had tended to place strong emphasis on the recruiting process and to assume that the interviewing process would take care of itself. They were shocked and horrified to hear that nursing candidates perceived their hospitals' interviewers as rude and abrupt. They decided to "modify the product" in the following ways:

- Make sure that all interviewers were the warmest and most enthusiastic managers around.
- Make sure that each interviewee had an opportunity to meet with a peer, namely, a young Alpha Hospital nurse who had graduated within the past two years.
- Interviewers were given much more intensive training than they had been given before, along with practice sessions and role playing. In the training they were encouraged to emphasize the positioning of the hospital—that is, its stability and financial security—throughout the interview.
- Each interviewee received a small, tasteful gift.

During the focus group, as noted, participants said that some of Alpha Hospital's recruitment ads were "too cutesy." They also gave other specific recommendations for future ads. These reactions provided valuable input to the human resources department at Alpha. They worked with their advertising agency to design ads that were more consistent with the participants' tastes.

In summary, it is clear that recruiting nurses is not the same thing as selling a product or service. However, various marketing tools can be applied to the problem in a helpful way. The key to applying a marketing approach to any problem lies in remembering the definition of marketing.

Understanding the Customers' Needs

The three basic types of market research that are used in industry have also been applied usefully in health care settings. They are focus groups, surveys, and personal interviews.

Focus Groups. Let's say that you want to renovate and improve your maternity services and that you want to get some customer input before you begin this expensive and time-consuming process. A good approach to the problem would be to use a focus group.

First, you would recruit eight to ten members of your target audience to be participants. (There are companies that will recruit participants for you if you do not wish to do it yourself.) Then you would select a focus group leader or moderator. This could be a professional moderator or a sensitive, empathetic member of the hospital staff.

The job of the moderator is to encourage the participants to be relaxed and comfortable, so that they are willing to share their attitudes and opinions candidly in a group setting. The moderator asks questions of the participants, based on a discussion guide. The discussion guide consists of questions that have been created by management with the objective of obtaining valuable customer input in the focus-group setting.

It is very important that the focus-group participants discuss their views in a nonthreatening atmosphere. For this reason, the typical situation is that only the moderator is in the room with the participants. Since management people are not in the room, they can learn the results of the focus-group discussion in a variety of ways. First, they can conduct the session in a specially designed focus-group facility. These facilities are frequently tucked away in shopping malls, and are equipped with one-way mirrors, so that management can observe the discussion unobtrusively. (Naturally, participants must be advised that they are being observed before the session begins.) In the vast majority of cases, participants do not find such scrutiny disturbing or inhibiting.

Second, management can learn the results through videotaping or audiotaping. A third, but least preferred, way is to have the moderator take notes, but this may distract her or him from leading the group discussion.

Focus groups are valuable in any situation in which you need to obtain rich, qualitative data from customers. Here are some examples:

- Hospital management wants to get an in-depth evaluation from discharged patients as to how they felt about the wide variety of services and personnel that they were exposed to.
- The director of a substance abuse rehabilitation service wants to know why service agencies — their key referral sources — are not making referrals as they used to.
- A nursing vice president wants to get an in-depth understanding of what motivates recently graduated nursing students to select one hospital over another.
- A hospital advertising director has three different possible ads to promote the hospital's new physician referral service. She wants to solicit customer evaluation before deciding which ad to select.

The greatest value of focus groups is that they permit management to obtain rich, in-depth attitudes and opinions from customers. Frequently, focus-group discussions will come up with valuable information that management would not even have thought of soliciting. For example, in a recent focus group, participants spontaneously volunteered that they perceived the hospital to be a for-profit organization. Although it never occurred to the hospital that this misperception could exist, the information is quite valuable at a time when hospitals' nonprofit status is being questioned. As a result the hospital included a tag line indicating its nonprofit status on all subsequent advertising and communications.

The main limitation of focus groups is the restricted number of participants. Obviously one cannot generalize specific findings from a focus group to the population at large. For example, one cannot say that because five out of ten focus-group participants prefer a certain hospital, then 50 percent of all consumers will prefer that hospital.

Surveys. Many people are familiar with telephone interviews through their own personal experience as respondents. Almost everyone has had the experience of being called on the telephone and asked, "Would you kindly take a moment to answer some questions about a new banking service we are thinking of offering?" or "Will you please answer some questions about the toothpaste that you use?" Telephone interviews are used when more quantitative information is required. A hospital that wishes to predict the percentage of individuals in its service area who would sign up for a fitness program could gain such information via telephone interviews. A five-minute survey conducted among 200 to 300 area consumers would provide a good basis for estimating future utilization of the program.

Mail surveys are frequently used when telephone interviews are too difficult to conduct or too expensive. For example, physicians may be difficult to reach for a telephone survey, but may be more likely to respond to a well-designed mail survey.

Personal Interviews. These are used infrequently in health care research because the cost of professional interviewers usually is beyond the research budget of health care marketers.

Conclusion

A marketing mindset and astute application of marketing strategies can help health care organizations better meet people's health care needs and, in so doing, strengthen the organization's competitive position. Also, marketing strategies can help nursing professionals address the compelling challenges that face the nursing profession and your own nursing service's position as the provider of choice for nurses and nursing care.

The key: Marketing needs to be understood as more than the sum of its parts. It is not advertising. It is not pricing. It is not sales. It is an integrated planning and decision-making process that involves (1) finding out what the customer wants and needs, and (2) fulfilling those needs better than anyone else while (3) meeting your financial objectives.

References

Kotler, P. *Marketing Management.* (5th ed.) Englewood Cliffs, N.J.: Prentice Hall, 1984.

Tilbury, M. A., and Fisk, T. A. *Marketing and Nursing.* Owings Mills, Md.: National Health Publishing, 1989.

CHAPTER 3

Designing
Effective Organizations

Lawrence G. Hrebiniak

This chapter will discuss the design of effective organizations, with the emphasis on *effective*. Decades ago, it was suggested that effectiveness in this context denotes an organization "doing the right things." It is goal oriented. It indicates that the organization is serving its clients well and implies a market orientation. Although cost or efficiency clearly must enter into managers' decision making, effective organizations are not concerned solely with the low-cost production of services, but rather with their impact or efficacy in the intended market. Goals or desired outcomes are the primary drivers of decision making; cost and related concerns, while important, constitute secondary supportive decisions, that is, how to achieve effective care in the most efficient manner.

Why focus on this definition of organizational effectiveness? Organizations cannot survive without being effective, but they can survive if they are not efficient. Products or services that are differentiated in the mind of the consumer as in some way high quality or unique typically can demand a premium price, compensating for or negating some inefficiencies or higher costs. (Of course, gross inefficiencies or out-of-line high costs are another story.) Emphasizing effective performance as the fundamental element of organizational strategy and as a modus operandi is a necessary condition for performance in industries trying to capture a viable market share.

There are four critical ingredients in the design of organizations that will be both effective and sufficiently efficient to survive over the long term:

1. Sound strategy formulation and planning processes
2. Structure appropriate to the strategic thrust of the organization
3. A means of achieving effective coordination and integration, especially laterally, across function or skills
4. Incentives and controls that support the objectives and operating structure of the organization

Sound Strategy Formulation and Planning Processes

The development of sound strategic and short-term planning processes is the first step in designing effective organizations. The more important process is clearly the formulation of strategy because it focuses on the development of long-term objectives and the alignment of organizational capabilities and environmental contingencies. This focus on objectives and emphasis on "fit" between internal capabilities and external factors underlines the importance of effectiveness for organizations' growth. The essence of strategy formulation is analysis of the competition and the industry and/or portfolio, enabling the organization to direct and deploy its scarce resources and talents over time. Creation of a market or niche via strategic positioning is intended to reduce organizational vulnerability and enhance its prospects for survival. Because Chapter One has already dealt in depth with planning, suffice it to say that strategic and short-term planning are the critical first steps to ensure that organizations are "doing the right things."

Structure Appropriate to the Strategic Thrust of the Organization

The second step is to ensure that the organizational structure is appropriate to the strategic and operating tasks at hand. Structure may be simply defined as the way an organization groups and uses specialized human resources. Structure denotes "boxes and lines," with emphasis on both the formal configuration of functions, departments, or other "clusters" of people and the informal authority and influence patterns that result.

There are, of course, many ways to group and use specialized resources. The two building blocks of organizational structure that are prototypes and help explain other, more complex structural forms are process specialization and purpose specialization.

A structure based on *process specialization* is built around common functions, skills, or areas of expertise. It emphasizes the *parts* of an overall task, for example, the components of effective treatment of a patient. Whenever services are needed for this patient, they are drawn from the respective division that specializes in that service, such as dietary, pharmacy, laboratory, nursing, or finance. These specialties are centrally controlled and are available to anyone who needs them in the organization. The focus on common skills results in efficiency and/or cost reduction because of the economies of scale and the experience curve that specialists incur.

At the other extreme is "pure" *purpose specialization,* in which an organization is built around relatively self-contained units or teams, such as divisions, strategic business units, and product lines. Within each unit, resources exist to perform *all* the necessary tasks, minimizing coordination and integration costs and the need for interdependence. Because of the emphasis on self-containment and the consequent ability to focus on the task or client, purpose specialization often achieves effective performance. Its strength is its focus on "ends," or the needs of its clients, rather than on "means," or the processes it uses in common with other parts of the organization.

Of course, not all structural units can be classified as having "pure" types of specialization. Many organizations try to combine these two types of structural specialization into a structure that captures the best of both. The structural design task facing managers is how to combine process and purpose specialization in ways that achieve effective performance at reasonably efficient levels.

Consider an example of a small organization with one

product line and a three-part production process. The organizational structure is relatively simple. To produce the product (output), the three processes are coordinated by one general manager. When a second product line is introduced, the manager has two design alternatives. The first is to divide the organization structure into two departments based on purpose/product line. By not having to rely on centralized processes, scheduling and coordination problems are eliminated, and the ease of management and concentration of focus in the "purpose departmentalization" are obvious benefits. The second alternative is to structure the organization using "process departmentalization," creating separate, self-contained product lines for each division, duplicating the services and expertise in each division.

At the extreme of pure purpose specialization, each division would stand alone with its own staff and facilities. The two division managers can each focus on separate, differentiated tasks that lead to different market foci and effective outcomes appropriate to the particular product or client. There are two major costs potentially associated with this design option: (1) the loss of economies of scale because the separate functions are usually smaller in each division than they would be together and (2) the duplication of scarce resources in each division.

An alternative plan would retain the original structure of the organization around common processes or functions but would apply it to the two product lines. The manager's task is to coordinate the flow of work for the different product lines, using common facilities and enabling the component functions of the organization to specialize according to the processes that they perform. In a hospital example, inpatients and outpatients would use the same ancillary services, leading to economies of scale because of the greater volume, although they would otherwise be regarded as separate product lines. Fewer people would be needed in centralized functions, again leading to efficiencies.

Process specialization is, however, not without its problems. The increased need for coordination becomes more serious and more costly as the number of product lines increases. Emphasis on processes or means could obscure differences in clients or markets and the need to attend to end products. Also, all work is the same, repetitive and routinized, potentially leading to a distance from and a lack of concern for "real" clients, and thereby to a loss or dissipation of effective outcomes (ends).

In essence, there is a point at which the economic benefits of process specialization are outweighed by the costs of coordination and consequent loss of effectiveness. This often comes with growth — that is, the number of inpatients and outpatients grows so large as to make coordination burdensome. To avoid this problem, the manager can again combine purpose specialization with process specialization in a division structure. Each division is large and can reap economies of scale, and each can focus on its own product line, thereby increasing effectiveness, but each has enough volume also to be efficient. When organizational units grow large enough or when markets, customers, product lines, or geographic areas are well defined, the organization can reincorporate process departmentalization into purpose specialization by creating a division with functional subunits.

Ultimately, the choice of structure is dictated by strategy and competitive conditions. Under perfectly competitive conditions the economies or efficiencies of process specialization may be critical. Under more typical conditions, purpose specialization may be required to serve different markets well, thereby achieving effectiveness. As organizations grow or change their strategic thrusts, different combinations of structural types will be required to meet important objectives and allow the organization to compete effectively.

A Means of Achieving Effective Coordination and Integration

The third step in designing effective organizations is to ensure that coordination or integration is well done. Effectiveness implies a unity of effort around a common and clear purpose, achieved by sound coordination processes. Integrating mechanisms are especially important in those areas where experts specialize on only part of an entire process. Each function focuses on its own specialized task (for example, lab personnel do lab work, the dietary group does its job) rather than on the need for coordinating tasks to solve a particular (patient's) problem.

Conflicts that may develop because of homogeneity within task groups versus heterogeneity among groups make effective coordination even more necessary to achieve organizational goals. People rarely see problems as arising from their own or their group's mistakes, but find it easy to assign blame to personnel in other areas (for example, manufacturing is to blame because it failed to do what engineering specified, or the medical staff is to blame because it gave incomplete instructions to the nursing staff). Again, coordination of efforts across the different units whose personnel are involved but who may have a different perspective is critical to effective performance. There are a number of ways to achieve this coordination, ranging from relatively simple direct personal contact to very complex matrix organizations. How the formal structure relates to the informal role of the individuals within it depends on coordination. The matrix, an operating structure that stresses lateral coordination, could not work without effective integrators, teams, and two-boss managers to coordinate the desires and needs of different units. One method of achieving integration is hierarchial coordination, involving reliance on rules, performance programs, and standardized procedures. Hierarchical coordination is most feasible when tasks are relatively simple. As tasks become more complex, standard procedures or responses become inadequate, and it is necessary to provide for more lateral coordination. In the typical matrix organization employees from certain departments or functional areas perform services for a "project" or unit for a period of time. They become part of a team. They work for two supervisors. They must meet the demands of the project or unit manager while simultaneously meeting the demands of the functional manager. They must frequently coordinate and solve conflicts across units with divergent demands or performance criteria.

The matrix, then, stresses both horizontal and vertical communication. It is a "purpose" organization superimposed on a "functional" or "process" organization. Functional people can be moved to projects to solve problems as they arise. Emphasis is placed on getting the right people to solve the problem without referring it up the organization. There is bilateral dependence between project and function in the matrix. Division managers depend on the expertise of functional personnel; functional managers expect division managers to use their employees' time and skills and justify their existence in the organization. In our hospital example each case in the division of inpatient services is managed as a separate project. Services of a patient-care team of specialized employees, each of whom is drawn from a department in the hospital with its own director, are ordered and directed by the case manager. There is bilateral dependence, and a superordinate goal (quality care) exists to integrate the system and guarantee effective performance. Team members bring their own expertise to the problem, and because they need not pass information on to superiors and wait for a decision, treatment is more timely. Team decision making is also more suited to complex tasks in which no one person can alone collect sufficient information to be able to make an effective decision. Finally, the existence of the many perspectives of the team members helps to ensure that concerns are aired and political problems avoided. Teams are not free of conflict, but they can coordinate the work of diverse kinds of employees for the benefit of the client.

In sum, complex organizations need to develop methods of achieving coordination if they are to perform effectively. There are many ways to achieve this integration, ranging from simple, direct contact among players to hierarchical coordination, and finally to more complex structures such as matrix organizations. Whichever methods are employed, the goal is to achieve a unity of effort around common objectives and whatever criteria define effective organizational performance.

Incentives and Controls

The final step in designing effective organizations is the development of an appropriate system of incentives and controls. These can be highly related or interdependent; incentives motivate desired performance, while controls ensure that performance is consistent with desired ends. Controls, by providing feedback about performance, add the much-needed capacity for flexibility and ability to change as organizations adapt over time.

To ensure effective performance, incentives must be attached to important goals or outcomes. They should motivate the specifically desired performance, and care must be taken to ensure that they support both short-term and strategic objectives. Thus to hope for quality-of-care improvements over a five-year term while rewarding only efficiency and cost reduction in the near term can spell disaster and produce major conflicts within the organization.

Similarly, incentives should not fuel or exacerbate conflicts between or among organizational units. Rewarding medicine or the laboratory for one type of performance while rewarding nursing for a performance with conflicting objectives only creates confusion and animosity within the organization. Care must be taken to select the right behavior to reward, as it is foolish to seek a particular outcome while at the same time rewarding another. A classic example is where universities reward faculty with tenure or promotion solely on the basis of publications, although they repeatedly say that they value good teaching. Faculty members quickly and accurately recognize what administration really thinks about the importance of teaching and working with students. Similarly, if only high-admitting physicians receive favors from the hospital administration, statements regarding the importance of any goals other than patient turnover and cash generation are likely to fall on deaf ears.

Incentives must be tied to clear, measurable indicators of performance. Rewarding individuals in purely subjective or capricious ways is both dangerous and motivationally debilitating. Desired performance must be measurable, able to be operationalized, and unambiguous. If "enhancing morale" or "improving quality care" is important, the variables or proxy measures for those ends must be unequivocal and able to be articulated. Only then can incentives be effectively tied into varying levels of performance. Good performance can only be recognized and rewarded if it is absolutely clear how one is going to know whether it occurs.

In essence, *incentives tell people what to do*. They inform individuals as to what is important to the organization. They are central to motivation and must fit the organizational culture within which they are employed.

Control follows logically from the planning process that determined (1) objectives and (2) the incentives needed to support them. Objectives and incentives motivate and provide direction; controls monitor and follow up performance to determine if actual behavior is consistent with intentions. The control process tracks performance and provides the feedback necessary to evaluate results and take any needed corrective action.

This process is dependent on the comparison of actual performance and objectives or desired performance. Tracking actual performance against objectives or milestones initiates the control process by inquiring whether there is a deviation between what is being aimed at (desired) and what is accomplished (actual performance). Responding to deviations between actual and desired levels of achievement (for example, between budgeted and actual cash flows) represents what is commonly referred to as *management by exception*.

The identification and follow-up of exceptions or deviations between actual and desired performance provides an important evaluative aspect of the control process. Understanding the significance of these deviations, their causal or contributing factors, and the variables underlying and explicating them facilitates organizational learning and provides the ability to plan in the future. The process of evaluation and learning is critical for continued success and organizational effectiveness.

Formal appraisal procedures must also measure performance against objectives. Review mechanisms should compare actual against desired levels of achievement and formal feedback, and rewards should depend to some degree on the results of this review. Evaluation and feedback are central to the control process and are critically important for the reinforcement of behavior that is consistent with effective performance criteria.

Finally, something of consequence must result from the process of control and the comparisons, analysis, and evaluation it implies. Included should be rewards for outstanding performance, necessary changes in objectives or plans and other corrective actions, and development of alternative, more timely sources of information to facilitate tracking and evaluation of performance. It is critical that the process of evaluation and follow-up not contribute to an unhealthy emphasis on avoiding risks and errors at any cost. Rigid and uncompromising control systems that do not tolerate error breed an overly conservative emphasis on maintaining the status quo, with a debilitating effect on motivation as well as on the formulation and achievement of plans of action.

Control clearly makes many essential contributions to designing effective organizations. It guarantees that the right performance criteria are being achieved and allows the necessary flexibility and follow-up that will ensure that the organization continues to "do the right things." Most important, control enables the organization to learn from past performance, thereby strengthening its ability to plan for the future. It represents the final critical step in the process of designing effective organizations.

References

Galbraith, J. *Designing Complex Organizations.* Reading, Mass.: Addison-Wesley, 1973.

Hrebiniak, L. G., and Joyce, W. F. *Implementing Strategy.* New York: Macmillan, 1984.

Macmillan, I. C., and Jones, P. E. "Designing Organizations to Compete." *Journal of Business Strategy,* 1984, *4* (4), 11–26.

Van de Ven, A. H., and Joyce, W. F. (eds.). *Perspectives on Organizational Design and Behavior.* New York: Wiley, 1981.

PART 2

Economic Issues and Support Systems

CHAPTER 4

Understanding the Economics of Health Care Decision Making

Mary Kaye Willian
John M. Eisenberg

Conducting economic analyses of health care services has become increasingly popular in the past decade for a variety of reasons. Passage of the Medicare Prospective Payment legislation in the mid 1980s focused attention on the rising costs of hospital services and put in place mechanisms that were intended to constrain inflation in this area (Medicare Prospective Payment Assessment Commission, 1989). As Congress considered legislation that would have mandated the private sector to provide certain benefits for employees, corporations have become increasingly concerned about the amount they are spending on health care and are seeking ways to reduce these expenses (Gabel, DiCarlo, Fink, and de Lessovoy, 1989; Moyer, 1989). Simultaneously, there has been a growing awareness that many medical services may be unnecessary and perhaps even harmful. Finally, documentation of geographic variations in medical practice has stimulated the health care community, policymakers, and others to seek a more thorough understanding of the impact of these differences on the costs of care (Brook and others, 1984; Chassin and others, 1986; Wennberg, 1986).

These factors, coupled with the nursing shortage of the 1980s, have mandated that the nursing profession look critically at its role in providing care in an efficient and effective manner. As a result, nursing executives are now evaluating all aspects of nursing and medical practice patterns, how they complement and supplement one another, and how each may directly or indirectly affect the economics of the other. Increasingly, both professional disciplines are recognizing that joint, as opposed to parallel, practices may be more economically efficient, effective, and perhaps even satisfying to the involved professionals. Initial research in this area indicates that effective collaboration between nurses and physicians results in higher-quality patient care (Draper, 1987; Knaus, Draper, Wagner, and Zimmerman, 1986).

In this chapter, we will introduce the basic concepts of economic analysis. We will describe the three major types of analysis, review the various categories of costs that may be included in such evaluations, and discuss other relevant issues, including assessment of costs versus charges and the role of discounting in economic studies. Throughout the presentation, these concepts will be applied to clinical decisions that nurses may face in their health care practices. We hope that these conceptual tools and techniques will be useful to nurses in their clinical and managerial responsibilities for decision making to produce better results in terms of patient care, treatments, and programs.

Basic Economic Principles

In assessing the costs of health care practice, it is important first to understand the distinction between the often used but equally often misused terms *efficacy* and *effectiveness*.

Determination of Cost. Efficacy examines whether a specific type of care *can* work; it raises the question of whether the therapy or program produces more positive than negative results to those individuals who fully comply with the treatment protocol or program. Effectiveness refers to whether the therapy or program *does* work; it raises the question of whether the therapy or program produces more positive than negative effects when extended to the general population. Efficacy is tested under ideal circumstances, while effectiveness is examined under real-world or clinical conditions in which numerous uncontrolled influences may impinge on the results.

To clarify this point, consider the introduction of a new drug delivery system for hospitalized patients. This system, when tested under ideal conditions, was shown to deliver the drug more accurately and efficiently than the traditional method of administration. However, in the hospital setting, the nurses believed that it was cumbersome to use because of its design. They also found that they pushed the device harder against the patient's skin during administration, resulting in bruises, and that they monitored the patient more closely because they were unsure whether the patient actually received the drug. Thus, while the system proved to be efficacious in an ideal setting, it was not effective in the real clinical world (Willian and Koffer, 1989). To illustrate this point further, assume that a new cholesterol-lowering agent is introduced that has proved to be efficacious in clinical trials but causes annoying though not life-threatening side effects, resulting in poor patient compliance. While the drug's efficacy has been documented in the ideal setting of a controlled trial, it will not be effective if patients refuse to take it.

Two other concepts that should be considered in an economic analysis are *efficiency* and *equity*. Efficiency raises the question of what the service costs compared with its benefits. While the drug delivery system just described may, in fact, deliver a more accurate dose of insulin, it may be too costly for everyday clinical practice. That is, providers and the health care system, after weighing the costs and benefits, may be willing to tolerate a 0.5 percent dosage error in exchange for a less costly system.

Equity addresses the problem of distributing resources in a fair manner to those in need. The best technological advance is worth little if it does not reach those who need it. Consider the example of mammography screening. Until passsage of the Medicare Catastrophic Coverage Act, which extended payment for this screening procedure, it was available to all beneficiaries but actually was accessible only to a very specific segment of the population (Christensen and Katsen, 1988). Those who had the finances to pay out of pocket could obtain the examination, but low-income beneficiaries with limited resources may not have been able to afford it. There was, therefore, inequitable distribution of this health care resource.

Nurse executives are faced with the important question of resource allocation whenever decisions are being made about the implementation of a new program within their institution. Who will it be offered to, how much will be charged, and how frequently in the course of care will it be used? This same decision-making process should also be undertaken when a service or program is deleted. Who is left uncovered, where will services be obtained, and can patients afford the alternative provider?

Definitions of Cost

Cost is defined by most economists as the consumption of a resource that otherwise could have been used for another purpose. Once the resource has been used, the opportunity to employ it for another purpose has been lost. Therefore, its value in the next-best use (now no longer possible) is called its *opportunity cost*. For example, if a hospital has only one treatment course of a drug left available, the opportunity to use it is lost once it has been administered to a patient. When a dollar is used to purchase a health care service, the money has been spent and cannot be recovered. When deciding to use a new device or drug or to implement a new program, clinical and management decision makers need to consider what options they are foregoing.

There are several different categories of costs that may be considered in an economic analysis: direct, indirect, and intangible. It may not be possible or even desirable, depending on the study's perspective, to measure all categories in one study, but to the extent possible it is important to identify the most relevant ones.

Direct Costs. Direct costs represent monetary transactions and may include expenditures for medical or nonmedical products and services. Direct medical costs usually include those of hospitalization, drugs, laboratory tests, radiological procedures, rehabilitation, durable medical equipment, and nursing services. These costs are relatively easy to identify and often straightforward to measure, and they may be thought of as the resources used in the provision of care. These are the costs that constitute the half-trillion dollars spent on medical care each year in the United States (Levit and Freeland, 1988). However, the direct medical costs of a new drug administration system include not only supplies but also the time it takes pharmacy and nursing to prepare and administer the agent.

Direct nonmedical costs do not include the purchase of health care services but rather involve expenses for such illness-related items as food, transportation, lodging, special clothing, and home health nurses. Because these costs are rarely covered by insurance, they may have a significant impact on a family's finances, as documented by a study of children with cancer that found that almost one-fourth of the families' incomes was devoted to nonmedical out-of-pocket expenses (Lansky and others, 1979).

Indirect and Intangible Costs. In addition to direct medical and nonmedical costs, another category that has substantial economic impact is indirect costs. Indirect costs are those that occur because of loss of life or livelihood resulting from morbidity or mortality. Indirect morbidity costs may occur because of absence from work, decreased earning ability when working, or long-term disability, which necessitates a change in type of work. These production losses are also often considered a cost of the treatment or program, and the recovery of productivity from successful health care represents an economic benefit. Indirect mortality costs are, in essence, the costs of premature death, which may be calculated in two ways: the human-capital and the willingness-to-pay approaches (Landefeld and Seskin, 1982; Rice and Hodgson, 1982; Rice, Hodgson, and Kopstein, 1985).

The human-capital approach involves the calculation of a person's net percentage value of the future stream of lifetime earnings that could have been expected had the individual not died prematurely. The individual's value then is determined by the person's future earning capacity. Although the technique is a relatively easy one to apply, it raises a number of problems.

For one, with this technique any group of people who have a lower expected income than another group will have a reduced calculated value for their stream of lifetime earnings. The elderly are a prime example, for they would be shown, by use of this method, to be worth little, if anything, because they expect minimal income from labor. Acton (1976) also emphasizes that, even if we could be satisfied that this method is conceptually sound, an important practical issue needs to be addressed: Market earnings may not equal the productivity of a person's labor. This may occur for numerous reasons, including the fact that some groups may face discrimination in their earnings due to race, ethnicity, or gender. In contrast, other people may be receiving income that is substantially greater than their productivity. Unless these potential distortions are taken into account, the human-capital approach may bias the use of resources, treatments, and programs to the preferences of higher-income groups.

In addition, the human-capital method is quite sensitive to the rate at which dollars in the future are handled. This concept is known as *discounting* and will be discussed more thoroughly later in the chapter. With a higher discount rate, the value in today's dollars is lower. This methodological detail can have a profound effect on calculating costs or benefits that may accrue in the distant future. Consider, for example, the implication for a preventive service, for which the cost is incurred today and is counted at full cost but for which the benefit is delayed and must be discounted substantially. Childhood immunizations and smoking-prevention programs are examples of programs in which the expenditure for the service is immediate but whose benefits may not be realized for several years. With discounting, the economic advantages of such programs would likely appear unattractive because the future benefits may be discounted substantially.

Because of these problems with the human-capital approach, many experts have suggested an alternative for valuing mortality and morbidity, the willingness-to-pay method. This approach is based on the fundamental assumption that an individual's preferences or priorities should be taken into account and that the value of these preferences and priorities can be expressed in monetary units. This approach, which is favored by many economists (especially those of the neoclassical school), attempts to simulate the marketplace in valuing health outcomes. The willingness-to-pay approach suggests that any outcome, such as a life lost or an organ removed, can be valued by the amount that someone would be willing to pay to avoid having the adverse event occur. These values are usually measured by asking people hypothetical questions framed in terms of lotteries, trade-offs, or scales (Patrick, Bush, and Chen, 1973; Torrance, 1987; Weinstein and Stason, 1977).

The willingness-to-pay approach may be used to value the productivity lost owing to mortality and morbidity as well as the less tangible outcomes of pain, suffering, and grief associated with the therapy or treatment. However, a major problem with this approach is that people generally have difficulty estimating their willingness to pay for hypothetical events, primarily because of major conceptual difficulties with handling such probabilities as dying prematurely or living out their lives with a handicap or vague or intangible outcomes that are difficult to quantify, such as pain and suffering (Kahneman and Tversky, 1973). Even if they can make these estimates, people will probably be willing to pay more if they have more income or resources. If the selection of health care programs were based principally on their preferences, this socioeconomic group would have an excessive influence on policy (Thompson, Read, and Liang, 1984).

Because these indirect and intangible costs (and benefits) of health care and of illness are so difficult to quantify, they are often not included in economic studies. If they are included, the human-capital approach is usually used to quantify indirect costs of mortality and morbidity.

Other Cost Issues

One of the chief problems in economic analyses is the use of inadequate or inappropriate proxy measures in an attempt to attain "true" costs. Frequently, market prices such as hospital billing or insurance data are used as surrogates for "true" costs.

Cost and Charges. In the calculation of direct costs it is important to remember that charges are not the same as costs, for they are often set by the marketplace or by regulation (Finkler, 1982). In addition, charges do not differentiate between fixed and variable costs. Since fixed costs usually include overhead, they must be allocated among the various services that are provided. Charges may also cross-subsidize other products or services. For example, in some hospitals, charges for pharmaceuticals may help support services for which bills are not rendered, such as nursing or social services.

In making determinations of costs, it is important to distinguish those that are fixed and do not change (at least in the short term) with the volume of services provided from those that are variable and will change with the level of output. For example, the purchase of a computerized nursing patient classification system would be considered a fixed cost whereas the nurses' time and the supplies used to implement the system would be variable.

A second example would be resources used by patients staying an additional day in the hospital. Nursing costs, in this instance, would be considered fixed (in the very short term), because the extra day is likely not to be demanding of nursing services, and additional personnel are usually not added. The fee for the payer's physician visit, on the other hand, would be considered variable (from the payer's perspective), because the visit probably would not have been made unless the patient were in the hospital.

The Discount Rate. The costs and outcomes of a health care program or treatment rarely occur entirely in the same time period. More often than not they are incurred over several months or years. To deal with these discrepancies in time, discounting is used. The concept of discounting deals with the fact that a cost or an outcome today is not equivalent in value to the same cost or outcome in the future. In general, most people would prefer to have something today instead of having it in the future, and if they have to wait, they would want more to compensate for the delay. Another way to present this concept is to say that current dollars are worth more than future dollars. In order to take time into account, discounting is used in an attempt to make them the same value.

The discount rate selected, however, will have a substantial impact on the results (Keeler and Cretin, 1983). When a treatment's benefits are deferred, the use of a lower discount rate will make such a program appear more cost effective than if a higher rate were selected. Table 4.1 illustrates this point. Assume that Program X represents a cancer treatment project in which benefits will be realized within a five-year period, and Program Y involves a preventive health project (for instance, cholesterol reduction) initiated in childhood with the benefits realized in adulthood. If there is no discounting or if a 2 percent rate is used, Program Y proves most cost beneficial, but the reverse is true if the 4 percent rate is selected.

Table 4.1. Example of the Effect of
Discount Rate on Program Ranking.

	Year			Sum ($) at Discount Rate		
	0	*5*	*20*	*0%*	*2%*	*4%*
	Program X					
Benefits ($)	0	125,000	0	125,000	113,216	102,741
Costs ($)	100,000	0	0	100,000	100,000	100,000
Net benefit ($)				25,000	13,216	2,741
	Program Y					
Benefits ($)	0	0	200,000	200,000	134,594	91,278
Costs ($)	100,000	0	0	100,000	100,000	100,000
Net benefit ($)				100,000	34,594	− 8,722

Source: Reprinted with permission from Kenneth E. Warner and Bryan R. Luce, *Cost-Benefit and Cost-Effectiveness Analysis in Health Care: Principles, Practice, and Potential* (Ann Arbor, Mich.: Health Administration Press, 1982), p. 97.

Which discount rate to select stimulates vigorous debate among economists and economics researchers. The market interest rate is frequently used as a reference point. Today, discount rates of 5 to 6 percent are often used. The careful reader of economic analyses should determine whether costs as well as benefits have been discounted and should pay attention to the rates that are used.

The role of time is also important in economic analysis because of the possibility that additional costs (or savings) may be incurred subsequent to the clinical decision being analyzed. For example, if a treatment causes a delayed adverse outcome, the costs of that outcome should be counted as a "downstream" cost. It is clearly an induced cost (or savings), one that would not have occurred were it not for the immediate intervention. For example, if angioplasty is performed, the likelihood of the need for a repeat procedure in subsequent years should be taken into account.

Types of Economic Studies

It is important to know that there are different types of economic studies and to understand their relative strengths and weaknesses. These types include cost-identification analysis, cost-effectiveness analysis, and cost-benefit analysis.

Cost-Identification Analysis. Here the question "What is the cost?" is asked. By calculating the costs incurred because of a disease or because of the health services used to treat it, the cost of alternative ways of providing care can be determined. This measurement is expressed in terms of the cost per service provided. For example, one might calculate the dollars spent per case treated or per additional test or treatment provided.

Cost-identification analysis is called by some experts *cost-minimization analysis* because it may be used to identify the lower or lowest cost of various diagnostic or therapeutic strategies. Its central assumption is that the outcomes of the strategies being considered are equivalent. The goal is to find the least expensive way of achieving the outcome.

For example, one cost-identification study evaluated the savings from early hospital discharge of patients with osteomyelitis, followed by outpatient antibiotic treatment (Eisenberg and Kitz, 1986). The total costs of care for conventional inpatient treatment were $2,781 versus $2,271 for early discharge treatment, demonstrating a potential savings of $510 per patient. This study clearly illustrates the types of costs that may be included in such an analysis. As displayed in Table 4.2, all three categories in their analysis—direct medical and nonmedical as well as indirect costs—have been included by the authors.

Table 4.2. Types of Costs.

Direct		Indirect
Medical	*Nonmedical*	
Physician visits	Child care	Wages lost from work
Hospital costs	Home care	
Drugs and supplies	Transportation	
Ancillary services		

Source: Data extracted from Eisenberg and Kitz, 1986.

A cost-identification analysis may also be carried out to quantify the economic burden of a disease or its treatment. Eisenberg and his coauthors (1987), for example, found that the use of aminoglycoside antibiotics and the resulting nephrotoxicity in some patients produced a mean total additional cost of $2,501 per case of nephrotoxicity. To date, most clinical economic studies have focused on medical decision making and practice, not nursing decision making and practice and not the effects of medical practices on nursing time and costs. Inclusion of nursing in the equation is important, particularly since nursing personnel account for a major portion (approximately 50 percent) of a hospital's nonphysician labor budget. One of the few economic studies focusing on nursing emphasizes this point (Institute of Medicine, 1983).

Kitz and colleagues (1989), using the industrial techniques of time and motion analysis, compared the effects of using controlled versus noncontrolled oral analgesic agents for hospital inpatients. Not including the time and labor costs for taking inventory of controlled agents, these agents generated $1.84 in nursing costs compared with $0.53 for noncontrolled drugs. It was estimated that the annual savings the hospital would accrue by substituting noncontrolled for controlled oral agents on the three nursing units studied would amount to $34,427.

As useful as cost-identification analysis may be in determining the cost of health care or the financial burden of disease, it does not evaluate what these expenditures buy in terms of health outcomes. Thus, cost-identification analysis can guide health care practice only if a service has both lower cost and better or equal outcomes than its alternatives.

Cost-Effectiveness Analysis. A cost-effectiveness study goes a step beyond cost identification by incorporating both costs and outcomes in its analysis. It measures the net cost of providing a service (expenditures minus savings) as well as the outcomes or consequences. Outcomes are reported in a single unit of measurement, either a conventional clinical outcome (for example, years of life saved) or a measure that combines several outcomes on a common scale. The major advantage of a cost-effectiveness analysis is that it considers the possibility of improved outcomes in exchange for the use of more resources.

Investigators have developed several methods of converting disparate outcomes into a common scale, usually using the technique of utility analysis (Torrance, 1987; Torrance, Thomas, and Sackett, 1973; Weinstein and Fineberg, 1980). Utility analysis focuses on the quality of the health outcome produced by the treatment or therapy. It seeks to quantify the intangible outcomes. The utility or value of each outcome is measured in standardized units. These values can then be combined to yield an overall value or utility for the total impact of an intervention.

For example, the effectiveness of a treatment that improves both the duration and the quality of survival might be expressed in quality-adjusted life years (QALYs). Measurement of QALYs weighs years of life by the quality of those years, as determined by the presence of intangible outcomes such as disability. For example, five years of life with the morbid sequelae of a stroke might be equivalent to one year of life in perfect health, and thus equal to 1.0 QALY.

Cost-effectiveness analysis can be particularly helpful when considering policies recommending that clinicians and the public pursue certain clinical or health strategies. One study compared the cost-effectiveness of reducing serum cholesterol levels with three different therapies (Kinosian and Eisenberg, 1988). They found that the costs per year of life saved ranged from $17,800 for oat bran to $70,900 and $117,400 for cholestipol and cholestyramine, respectively. While significant national attention has been given to reducing serum cholesterol levels, policymakers and others have focused little on what the costs of implementing such a treatment program would be.

Hatziandreu and colleagues (1988) studied the cost-effectiveness of jogging as a health promotion activity. Using prevention of coronary heart disease events as the measure of outcome, the researchers found that the cost per quality adjusted life year gained was $11,313. The direct costs included such factors as jogging equipment, treatment of disease, and death. Indirect costs measured were exercise time and amount of time and, as a result, wages lost from work due to exercise injury or disability or death from coronary heart disease.

But what does this $11,313 figure mean? As with most economic analyses, it has little meaning unless it is compared with alternative therapies or treatments. In this case, the appropriate comparisons would be with other interventions to treat coronary heart disease, such as coronary artery bypass graft surgery ($40,000 for patients with mild angina) or the treatment of hypertension, with ranges from $25,000 to $65,000 depending on the severity of the disease.

For cost-effectiveness analysis to be pertinent to the concerns of patients and clinicians, the effect being measured needs to coincide with the stated objective. But whose objective, the patient's or the clinician's? The clinician may be concerned about the extension of life. Patients, on the other hand, may be more concerned about relief of pain and the resulting quality of their lives. Rarely have studies attempted to examine how these two perspectives may or may not coincide. The primary question in conducting such an analysis would be whether health care providers can serve as proxy decision makers for their patients.

Bunch and Chapman (1985) studied this issue in relation to individual preferences for methods of surgery for scoliosis and found striking concordance among the values of patients, family members, and surgeons. More research in this area needs

to be conducted to guide health care practitioners in selection
of therapies and treatments.

Cost-Benefit Analysis. Although cost-effectiveness analyses, including those in which the utilities of various outcomes
are measured, are useful to decision makers, they do not explicitly assess whether the outcomes are worth the cost. Cost-
benefit analysis — the third level of economic assessment of clinical practice — takes the analysis beyond measuring effectiveness
in clinical terms or abstract concepts of utility. Cost-benefit analysis forces a decision about whether the cost is worth the benefit
by measuring both in the same units. Since cost is usually measured in units of currency (in the United States, dollars), this
convention is retained in most clinical cost-benefit analyses.
While this form of analysis is theoretically appealing, it is often
restricted by measurement difficulties.

Two approaches are generally used to calculate the costs
and benefits and they may provide very different answers. With
the first approach, the net benefit or net cost is calculated by
subtracting the cost from the benefit. The second approach cal-
culates the ratio of benefits to costs. For example, suppose intervention A has a cost of $200 and a benefit of $300 and that
it can help one thousand people since it treats a common disease. The benefit-to-cost ratio is three to two, and the net benefit
of this intervention is $100,000 (that is, $300,000 – $200,000).
Intervention B has a cost of $100 and a benefit of $300, but
it helps only one hundred people. The benefit-to-cost ratio is
three to one — better than for intervention A — but the net benefit
is $20,000 (that is, $30,000 – $10,000). If one takes the general
view of the benefit to society, intervention A is preferred, since
its net benefit is larger. Use of the net benefit approach is usually
preferred to use of the benefit-to-cost ratio for reasons illustrated
with this example.

In a cost-benefit analysis of rubella vaccine, investigators
concluded that the economic benefits of the vaccination program
are greater if vaccine is offered once at age twelve to females
alone rather than to children of both genders at age six or less
(Schoenbaum and others, 1976). If rubella vaccination is to be

offered at age two or earlier, it is most cost beneficial to use combined measles and rubella vaccine. Including the direct and indirect costs of acute and congenital rubella that would be prevented, the benefit-to-cost ratio of monovalent vaccine for twelve-year-old females was 25 to 1, compared with 8 to 1 for two-year-old children of both genders.

Perspective of the Analysis

How does one decide which type of analysis to perform and the categories of costs to include in a clinical economic study? Establishing the perspective of the study, which should be done at the outset, helps make these decisions. Figure 4.1 demonstrates that there are several possible perspectives in an economic analysis of health care. Costs, outcomes, and benefits may be viewed differently by society, the patient, the payer, or the provider. For example, the cost to the payer, such as Blue Shield or Medicare, equals the charges that are allowed by that payer. However, the cost to the provider, such as a hospital, is the true cost of delivering the service, regardless of the charge (Finkler, 1982). The cost to patients, however, is the amount they pay for the service (that is, the portion not covered by insurance) plus the other costs that might be incurred because of illness or treatment, including time missed from work. The cost to society is the total net cost of all the other factors, including the patient's lost productivity and the expenses involved in the provision and receipt of health care.

Although many analysts have asserted that the social perspective is the proper perspective to take in an economic analysis, it is often instructive to carry out the analysis from more than one point of view. This makes it possible to identify conflicts. The previously cited example of an early discharge antibiotic program illustrates this dilemma (Eisenberg and Kitz, 1986). From the hospital's perspective this program saved money, but it increased costs for patients who usually bear the financial burden of home health services due to inadequate insurance coverage. As agents for their patients, physicians and nurses are then confronted with the ethical problem of whose interests

Figure 4.1. Considerations in Economic Analyses.

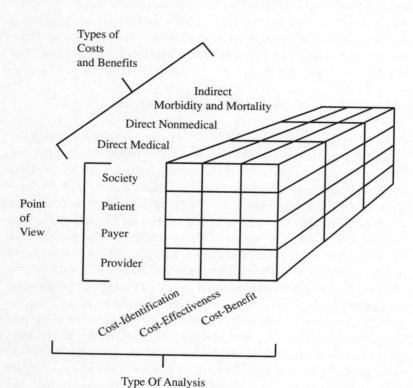

Type Of Analysis

Source: Adapted from Bombardier and Eisenberg (1985, p. 201).

take priority—their patients' or a sometimes financially strapped institution's. Resolution is not a straightforward or easy decision.

Conclusions

Some of the most important economic concepts and principles that are relevant to nursing and medical practice have been presented in this chapter. As executives, leaders in nursing are often faced with patient-care decisions that will be difficult, not only from an economic but also from an ethical perspective. To expand the repertoire of tools available in making these decisions and arriving at sound conclusions, the chapter has also introduced the concepts of clinical economic analysis. The responsibilities of the decision maker involve not only assessing the economic aspects of nursing practice but also evaluating how changes in other practices, such as those of medicine, pharmacy, and social work, will affect nursing practice and, of course, ultimately patient care.

However, a practical question remains: How does one decide which type of analysis to conduct? In making this decision the key considerations are the questions to be answered and the perspective to be taken. Although they are often viewed as the weakest research design, cost-identification (or cost-minimization) studies may be the most appropriate first step prior to undertaking a more complex and expensive cost-effectiveness or cost-benefit analysis. It may, for example, be sufficient to know the costs presently being incurred for a disease before the decision is made to proceed with developing a new drug or device. If expenditures are relatively low for a specific disease and the development costs moderate to high, dollars might be more effectively invested in another area. A second and more practical reason to select cost-identification analysis is that data may not be available to proceed with a cost-effectiveness or cost-benefit analysis.

Most users of economic analysis would prefer, however, to have an evaluation of what they are getting for their expenditures, and therefore would prefer that the more difficult utility analysis be used when quality of life is an important outcome, when combining both mortality and morbidity measures into one unit, or when the treatments or programs being compared have a wide range of different outcomes (Drummond, Stoddart, and Torrance, 1987).

Cost-benefit analysis, while theoretically the most desirable and useful of the three categories, is problematic to carry out in practice because it is difficult to reach consensus regarding the value to attach to the outcome measures such as a human life. Nevertheless, if agreement can be reached about these measurements, this form of analysis should be used.

The adjectives *cost-effectiveness* and *cost-benefit* are frequently misused and not well understood. Many assume that they mean "inexpensive" and fail to move to the next necessary steps of evaluating the ratio of the dollars expended to the value obtained. Nevertheless, when used correctly, economic analysis is a systematic method on which decision makers can rely to assist them in the selection of efficient uses of their limited resources.

References

Acton, J. P. "Measuring the Monetary Value of Life-Saving Programs." *Law and Contemporary Problems,* 1976, *40,* 46–72.

Bombardier, C., and Eisenberg, J. M. "Looking into the Crystal Ball: Can We Estimate the Lifetime Cost of Rheumatoid Arthritis?" *Journal of Rheumatology,* 1985, *12,* 201–204.

Brook, R. H., and others. "Geographic Variations in the Use of Services: Do They Have Any Clinical Significance?" *Health Affairs,* 1984, *3,* 63–73.

Bunch, W. H., and Chapman, R. G. "Patient Preferences in Surgery for Scoliosis." *Journal of Bone and Joint Surgery,* 1985, *67-A,* 794–799.

Chassin, M. R., and others. "Variations in the Use of Medical and Surgical Services by the Medicare Population." *New England Journal of Medicine,* 1986, *314,* 285–290.

Christensen, S., and Katsen, R. "Covering Catastrophic Expenses Under Medicare." *Health Affairs,* 1988, *7,* 79–83.

Draper, E. A. "Effects of Nurse/Physician Collaboration and Nursing Standards on ICU Patients' Outcomes." *Current Concepts in Nursing,* 1987, *1,* 2–8.

Drummond, M. F., Stoddart, G. L., and Torrance, G. W. *Methods for the Economic Evaluation of Health Care Programmes.* Oxford, England: Oxford University Press, 1987.

Eisenberg, J. M., and Kitz, D. S. "Savings from Outpatient Antibiotic Therapy for Osteomyelitis: Economic Analysis of a Therapeutic Strategy." *Journal of the American Medical Association,* 1986, *255,* 1584–1588.

Eisenberg, J. M., and others. "What Is the Cost of Nephrotoxicity Associated with Aminoglycosides?" *Annals of Internal Medicine,* 1987, *107,* 900–909.

Finkler, S. A. "The Distinction Between Cost and Charges." *Annals of Internal Medicine,* 1982, *96,* 102–109.

Gabel, J., DiCarlo, S., Fink, S., and de Lessovoy, G. "Employer-Sponsored Health Insurance in America." *Health Affairs,* 1989, *8,* 116–128.

Hatziandreu, E. I., and others. "A Cost-Effectiveness Analysis of Exercise as a Health Promotion Activity." *American Journal of Public Health,* 1988, *78,* 1417–1421.

Institute of Medicine. *Nursing and Nursing Education: Public Policies and Private Actions.* Washington, D.C.: National Academy Press, 1983.

Kahneman, D., and Tversky, A. "On the Psychology of Prediction." *Psychology Review,* 1973, *80,* 237–251.

Keeler, E. B., and Cretin, S. "Discounting of Life-Saving and Other Nonmonetary Effects." *Management Science,* 1983, *29,* 300–306.

Kinosian, B. P., and Eisenberg, J. M. "Cutting into Cholesterol: Cost-Effective Alternatives for Treating Hypercholesterolemia." *Journal of the American Medical Association,* 1988, *259,* 2247–2254.

Kitz, D. S., McCartney, M., Kissick, J. F., and Townsend, R. J. "Examining Nursing Personnel Costs: Controlled Versus Noncontrolled Oral Analgesic Agents." *Journal of Nursing Administration,* 1989, *19,* 10–14.

Knaus, W. A., Draper, E. A., Wagner, D. P., and Zimmerman, J. E. "An Evaluation of Outcome from Intensive Care in Major Medical Centers." *Annals of Internal Medicine,* 1986, *104,* 410–418.

Landefeld, J. S., and Seskin, E. P. "The Economic Value of Life: Linking Theory to Practice." *American Journal of Public Health,* 1982, *72,* 555–556.

Lansky, S. B., and others. "Childhood Cancer: Nonmedical Costs of the Illness." *Cancer,* 1979, *43,* 403–408.

Levit, K. R., and Freeland, M. S. "Data Watch: National Medical Care Spending." *Health Affairs,* 1988, *7,* 124–136.

Medicare Prospective Payment Assessment Commission. *Medicare Prospective Payment and the American Health Care System: Report to Congress.* Washington, D.C.: Medicare Prospective Payment Assessment Commission, 1989.

Moyer, M. E. "Data Watch: A Revised Look at the Number of Uninsured Americans." *Health Affairs,* 1989, *8,* 102–110.

Patrick, D. L., Bush, J. W., and Chen, M. M. "Methods for Measuring Levels of Well-Being for a Health Status Index." *Health Service Research,* 1973, *8,* 224–245.

Rice, D. P., and Hodgson, T. A. "The Value of Human Life Revisited." *American Journal of Public Health,* 1982, *72,* 536–537.

Rice, D. P., Hodgson, T. A., and Kopstein, A. N. "The Economic Costs of Illness: A Replication and Update." *Health Care Financial Review,* 1985, *7,* 61–80.

Schoenbaum, S. C., and others. "Benefit Cost-Analysis of Rubella Vaccination Policy." *New England Journal of Medicine,* 1976, *294,* 306–310.

Thompson, M. S., Read, J. L., and Liang, M. "Feasibility of Willingness-to-Pay in Chronic Arthritis." *Medical Decision Making,* 1984, *4,* 195–215.

Torrance, G. W. "Utility Approach to Measuring Health-Related Quality of Life." *Journal of Chronic Diseases,* 1987, *40,* 593–600.

Torrance, G. W., Thomas, W. H., and Sackett, D. L. "A Utility Maximization Model for Evaluation of Health Care Programs." *Health Service Research,* 1973, *7,* 228–245.

Warner, K. E., and Luce, B. R. *Cost-Benefit and Cost-Effectiveness Analysis in Health Care: Principles, Practice, and Potential.* Ann Arbor, Mich.: Health Administration Press, 1982.

Weinstein, M. C., and Fineberg, H. V. *Clinical Decision Analysis.* Philadelphia: Saunders, 1980.

Weinstein, M. C., and Stason, W. B. "Formulations of Cost-Effectiveness Analysis for Health and Medical Practice." *New England Journal of Medicine,* 1977, *296,* 716–721.

Wennberg, J. E. "Dealing with Medical Practice Variations: A Proposal for Action." *Health Affairs,* 1986, *3,* 6–32.

Willian, M. K., and Koffer, H. Unpublished report. Philadelphia Association for Clinical Trials, 1989.

CHAPTER 5

The Foundations
of Financial Management

Steven A. Finkler

Financial management is an area of growing concern for nurses in management positions. The current environment for hospitals and other health care organizations is such that financial issues are becoming more vital for nurse managers, in their supervisory roles within nursing departments, as well as for nurse executives, in their organizational roles that extend beyond nursing departments.

This chapter gives an overview of the field of financial management. It provides a survey of the three main components of financial management: financial accounting, managerial accounting, and finance. Financial accounting is concerned with reporting the financial position of the organization and the financial results of its operations. Managerial accounting provides accounting data for internal decision making. Finance is a field that provides tools for the management of the financial resources of the organization.

The roles of each of these three fields are discussed in an effort to give the reader a better understanding of what financial management is all about. The chapter provides only surface treatment of a breadth of material. Its goal is to educate the reader regarding the nature of the financial management field. This will give the reader a better understanding of the existing types of tools of financial management that can be called on to provide information for decision making. It will also allow the reader to come to a better understanding of how financial issues affect the organization and to have a better ability to communicate more effectively with the organization's financial officers, chief executive officer, and board.

Financial Accounting

Financial accounting is the one branch of financial management that focuses more on the past than on the future. With the methods of financial accounting, financial information is recorded in a chronological fashion. This information is then summarized and provided to a variety of users via a financial report. The report supplies the reader with information on the current financial position of an organization and on the organization's results of operations. This information can be used by a bank to determine how safe a loan to the organization would be. It can be used by an investor or philanthropist to determine whether an investment in or donation to the organization is appropriate. It can be used by the board of trustees/directors of the organization and by its management to determine whether major actions are required, to help ensure that the organization survives and accomplishes its mission.

The Essence of Financial Accounting. Accounting systems are based on an underlying equality of assets and equities. Assets are valuable resources owned by the organization. Equities are ownership claims against those resources. Part of the total value of the assets of an organization is claimed by creditors. These claims by outsiders are referred to as *liabilities*. The remainder of the assets is owned by the owners of the organization. For-profit corporations are owned by stockholders, and the ownership value is referred to as the *stockholders' equity*. In not-for-profit organizations, the assets not due to outsiders are owned by the organization itself. This ownership value is referred to as the *fund balance*. Liabilities plus either stockholders' equity or fund balance equal the total equities of the organization. This total is always equal to the total assets, since the equities merely reflect the various claims on the assets of the organization. Generally, the term *fund balance,* rather than *stockholders' equity,* will be used in this chapter, because most readers are likely to work in not-for-profit organizations.

When an event that will have an impact on the finances of the organization occurs, that event, referred to as a *financial transaction,* must be recorded so that the impact of the event can later be summarized and reported. This recording is done by use of a journal. Just as an explorer might record a chronology of events for an expedition by making entries in a journal, the accountant records a financial chronology of events by making entries in a journal, commonly referred to as *journal entries.*

This original entry of information in a journal is often referred to as *double entry.* Double-entry accounting is a system designed to ensure that our financial records maintain the underlying equality of assets and equities. A financial event cannot change just one asset. If one asset were to increase while nothing else changed, our assets would no longer equal our equities. An asset increase will occur only if some other asset is reduced, or if an equity rises. For example, if we borrow money from a bank, our cash will rise, but so will our liability to repay the bank. Double-entry accounting merely requires that we record not only the increase in cash but also the increase in the liability to the bank.

The journal serves a valuable purpose in keeping track of the specific events as they occur. However, it is often useful to have a summary of the impact on one specific asset or equity of all the events that have taken place. For example, on any given day we might want to know how much cash we have or how much money we owe to suppliers. Because an organization may well have millions of journal entries in a year, we need some way of determining the current balance for an asset or equity without reviewing every recorded journal entry.

To accomplish this, the information from each journal entry is transferred (posted) to *ledger* accounts. A ledger is a collection of individual accounts, in which an account, quite simply, is anything we want separately to keep track of or keep account of. After recording an entire transaction in a journal, we would take each individual asset or equity involved and update the ledger information pertaining to those accounts. For example, if we borrow money from a bank, after recording the journal entry we would increase the balance in the cash account in our ledger and increase the balance in our liability ledger account.

Asset, liability, and fund balance (or stockholder equity) accounts are referred to as *permanent* accounts. The balance that we have in each of these accounts at the end of an accounting period such as a year is also the balance at the beginning of the next year. We can use the balance information at the end of the year to develop a *statement of financial position,* or *balance sheet.* This financial statement reflects the equality of assets and equities by showing, in some detail, the amount of each type of asset and liability. For example, the aggregate amount of cash, receivables, inventory, buildings, equipment, payables, and long-term debt would be shown. Fund balance is a residual that adjusts to ensure that assets do in fact equal total equities. This statement tells the reader the current financial position of the organization.

There are also several types of *temporary* accounts. Revenues and expenses are the most important temporary accounts. Revenues and expenses reflect changes in the fund balance related to the provision of goods and services to our patients. When we provide services and charge for them, we receive a valuable asset — usually either cash or the patient's (or third-party payer's) promise to pay cash. That promise takes the form of an account receivable. The organization or its owners claim ownership of that valuable asset. During the year that ownership claim on assets generated from current provision of goods or services is referred to as a *revenue.*

In the process of providing services we typically use up valuable assets. For example, we use up inventory and supplies, or we pay cash for labor services. That decline in assets reduces the assets available to be claimed by owners, and it is referred to as an *expense* during the year. At the end of the year, all the expenses are subtracted from the revenues to calculate the year's profit or loss. Profit and loss are sometimes referred to as *surplus* and *deficit,* respectively. This information is presented in a financial statement called an *income statement,* or *statement of profit*

and loss, or *activity statement,* or *statement of revenues and expenses.*
Unlike the balance sheet, which shows the organization's financial position at a point in time, this statement shows how successful the organization was over a period of time. Revenue and
expense are referred to as temporary accounts because each year
they start over with a zero balance. That allows us to see how
well our operations succeed each year, separately and distinctly
from any preceding or subsequent year.

The process of recording information in a journal and
then transferring the information to a ledger allows us to find
the balance in each asset, liability, revenue, expense, or fund
balance account at any point in time. We can then use the
balances to prepare the balance sheet and income statement,
which summarize perhaps millions of individual transactions
to present a picture of the current financial position and the
results of operations of the organization. This process is the essence of financial accounting. There are several other important financial statements that are useful in interpreting the financial status of an organization. And there are many problems
that arise in determining when and how to record financial transactions. However, all the rest of financial accounting is built
on this base.

Additional Financial Accounting Issues. With the basic
framework of financial accounting laid out, we can now address
a variety of issues that must be understood to help in interpreting the financial information generated by an organization such
as a hospital.

The information prepared is generated from the organization's own perspective. Accountants refer to this as the *entity
concept.* The books and records of the organization must be
segregated from those of any other individual or organization.
Thus, the financial statements that are prepared can be used
by internal managers, suppliers, creditors, industry associations,
and other users, all with the common understanding that the
statements reflect the organization itself rather than the financial affairs of its managers, its owners, or some other commin-
gled organization.

In not-for-profit organizations, the financial records of the organization are subdivided into separate *funds,* and an accounting method referred to as *fund accounting* is employed. Each fund is treated as a separate entity, hence separate records must be maintained to comply with the entity concept. Hospitals typically have a general unrestricted operating fund, a plant fund, in some cases an endowment fund, and special-purpose funds. Fund accounting gained widespread usage among not-for-profit organizations for two primary reasons. The first concerns restricted gifts. If a donor wishes a gift to be used for a particular purpose, donating that gift to a specific fund limits its use. For example, if money is given for a new building rather than for current operations, donating the money to the hospital's plant fund will ensure that objective. Second, funds allow for a clear separation of authority and control. To the extent that we feel that not-for-profit organizations are less closely supervised than for-profits, whose owners have a vested interest, fund accounting can help to prevent giving too much control to any one manager. Different fiduciaries can be placed in charge of different funds.

Fund accounting aroused considerable controversy in the 1970s and 1980s, partly as the result of accounting abuses. Most readers of financial statements place their main emphasis on the statements for the general unrestricted operating fund. However, it is possible to manipulate the reported results by having certain revenues bypass this main set of statements and be buried within the detail of the restricted funds. Given the advances in accounting systems during the twentieth century, there are many accountants, including the author of this chapter, who feel that the benefits of fund accounting are more than offset by the added complexity and other problems they generate. These accountants are advocating changes in accounting rules away from fund accounting.

In preparing financial statements, accountants follow accounting rules that are referred to as *generally accepted accounting principles* (GAAP). These principles are a dynamic set of guidelines that are promulgated by an independent body, the Financial Accounting Standards Board. This board issues statements on financial accounting standards, interpretations of financial accounting standards, and technical bulletins. Accountants of individual organizations are not required by law to follow GAAP. However, there are many reasons underlying the widespread adherence to this uniform body of rules.

Many organizations hire a certified public accountant (CPA) each year to audit their accounting record and to issue an opinion regarding the organization's financial statements. Most banks will not lend to an organization that does not have a set of financial statements audited by a CPA. Many associations, such as the American Hospital Association, require their members to have an annual audit. For-profit organizations with more than thirty stockholders are required by law to have an annual audit by a CPA. The CPA's audit determines whether the organization has in fact followed GAAP in the preparation of their financial statements, as well as testing the accuracy and completeness of the organization's financial records.

In giving their audit report, CPAs make clear note of whether or not the financial statements were prepared according to GAAP. As a result, organizations that are audited by CPAs almost invariably comply with GAAP requirements. Such requirements go well beyond the issue of whether fund accounting should be used. There are many technical rules requiring that one specific approach to accounting be taken. Other rules allow for a choice from among several alternatives, as long as the choice made is disclosed. Disclosure of choices, and of any significant information not contained in the financial statements themselves, is made through the use of a set of notes that accompany an audited set of financial statements. Often these notes contain vital information.

Even with the formalized body of rules, great care must be taken in interpreting financial statement information. For example, accounting rules require that assets be recorded at their cost, adjusted for depreciation. Thus, if a hospital owns a medical office building that was built twenty years ago for $10 million, that building may show up on the hospital financial statements at a value of perhaps $5 million after deducting depreciation taken over that twenty-year period. However, given inflation

in real estate over the last twenty years, the building may well
be worth $25 million. An audit report would make no note of
that discrepancy. The CPA gives an opinion only that the financial statements are prepared in accordance with GAAP. In turn,
GAAP requires that assets be recorded at their cost, adjusted
for depreciation. Accounting statements frequently do not show
assets at what they are truly worth.

The reason for this odd situation is that we have no very
good way of knowing exactly what something is worth unless
we sell it. Rather than speculate on true values, accounting rules
call for reliance on the cost, which is definitively known. Thus
one must be quite careful to seek knowledgeable interpretation
of financial statement information before relying on it.

Managerial Accounting

Managerial accounting is a field that focuses on generating financial information to aid managers in the process of planning the
activities of the organization and in controlling those activities
as they take place. Whereas financial accounting has a very specific set of rules (GAAP), which result in a very specific set of
reports (for example, balance sheet, income statement), managerial accounting has neither rules nor specific forms for reporting the results of the acounting calculations. Quite simply,
managerial accounting uses any approach to any financial analysis that will provide managers with information for improved
decision making.

Cost Accounting. A substantial portion of managerial
accounting is focused on issues of cost measurement and cost
behavior. The most basic function of cost accounting is the determination of the costs of running the organization. Cost information is essential because it allows the managers of the organization to find out whether revenues will be adequate for the continued survival of the organization. If costs turn out to exceed
revenues, the continued existence of the organization is threatened.

However, the specific type of cost information collected
varies tremendously from industry to industry. The informa-

tion collected can focus on the costs of running individual departments or on the costs of producing products or services. The information collected can be highly detailed or highly aggregated. An underlying feature of all cost accounting systems is the recognition that it costs money to collect information about costs. One should never spend more money on information than that information is worth.

Traditionally, health care organizations have been excellent at weighing the value of cost information and determining how much and what type of information will be "good enough." For example, in hospitals the primary cost of operating a laundry department is labor. And labor is much more highly related to the number of pieces of laundry than to the number of pounds of laundry. However, it is far easier to keep track of pounds than pieces. Hospitals have judged that the more refined information available from knowing how many pieces of each type of laundry are generated by each department is not worth the extra cost of collecting that information. Therefore, the costs of the laundry department are assigned to other departments on the basis of the number of pounds of laundry generated.

This "good enough" approach has been used throughout health care cost accounting. In hospitals it has resulted in systems that focus on the costs of departments rather than on the cost of treating individual patients. As a result, hospitals have excellent systems of "responsibility reporting." That is, hospital cost accounting allows a close association of costs with the departments in which they are incurred. Individual hospital managers can be held accountable for the direct costs of their departments. As a result, it is possible to monitor the performance of clinical line managers.

On the other hand, such cost accounting systems are particularly weak at telling us how much it costs to treat a given type of patient. In fact, hospital cost accounting creates a wide variety of cross-allocations or cross-subsidizations between patients. For example, depreciation is allocated on the basis of square feet. However, it costs substantially more per square foot to build an operating room than it does to build a medical bed. Therefore, by allocating depreciation using a set amount per square foot, we are overallocating cost to medical patients and underallocating cost to surgical patients.

Under a system that reimburses costs, this approach was "good enough." However, under prospective payments systems, specifically DRGs for Medicare patients, a specific amount is paid for a specific type of patient. Under such a system it becomes much more important to know how much cost is really being incurred to treat different types of patients. Survival depends on knowing the true profit or loss related to each type of patient. As a result, hospitals are now changing their cost accounting to focus more on "product costing." Refining calculations of the cost for patients in each DRG will be a major focus of hospital accountants in the future.

In the calculation of costs, one element that has received much attention in the past and that will continue to be important for all managers, not just cost accountants, is the basic dichotomy between fixed costs and variable costs. Fixed costs are those that are unlikely to change as the result of typical variations in workload levels. For example, if occupancy rises from 85 to 88 percent, the salary of the director of nursing services would not be likely to change. Variable costs, on the other hand, do change in direct proportion to the workload level.

This dichotomy is crucial because it results in a relationship between the volume of activity and the profitability of the organization. If patient revenues occur at a set rate per patient (as under the DRG system), adding additional patients will increase certain variable costs but will not increase fixed costs. If the revenue associated with each patient exceeds the variable costs, profits are enhanced by the addition of more patients. In fact, even if the average cost is such that the hospital is currently losing money on each patient, as long as revenue per patient exceeds variable costs, its profits will increase (or losses will decrease) as the patient volume increases.

One area of cost accounting, *break-even analysis,* focuses on this cost-volume-profit relationship. The techniques of this section of managerial accounting allow one to determine just how much volume is required in order to break even, or to attain any specific desired profit level.

Fixed- and variable-cost information is also very useful for projecting future costs of a current activity under conditions of changing volumes. For example, suppose that we anticipate a 10 percent rise in the number of operating room hours over the next year due to an increase in the number of cases. How much will operating room costs rise? The answer is not 10 percent. Clearly, some of the costs of the operating room are fixed. Those costs will not rise in response to an increase in volume, so the increase will be less than 10 percent. But how much less? The techniques of cost estimation allow one to use historical information to determine a department's fixed and variable costs, so that improved projections can be made.

Fixed- and variable-cost information is also useful in making nonroutine decisions. Should the hospital open a new service or expand an existing service? Should the hospital accept an offer made by an HMO for a guaranteed number of patients, but at a cut-rate price? These issues tend to be complex problems along a number of dimensions: power, politics, mission, and so on. However, accounting in this area can create particular misery for the decision maker. The problem is that there is no simple answer to what something costs. For example, suppose that a hospital chief executive officer (CEO) is paid a yearly salary of $100,000. What patients are benefiting from the CEO, and in what proportions? That is hard to determine, but it is clear that the cost must be allocated to the hospital's patients if an assessment of the cost of each patient is wanted. Thus, the CEO, like all other overhead items, becomes a cost that is allocated to the various departments and ultimately to the patients. If a new service is added, the patients for that service will be charged for a portion of the salary of the CEO.

Suppose, however, that with the allocation of a share of CEO salary and other fixed overhead costs, it does not make sense to offer the new service—it is too costly. Suppose further that without the allocation the service would be profitable. Whether or not to offer the new service is a perplexing question. It is, however, one of the topics that have received much attention in the cost accounting area. The CEO salary will be incurred whether we have the new service or not. It will not change if the new service is offered. Therefore, it is not a relevant cost in determining whether to go ahead. The new service should be offered because it is profitable if the overhead allocation is not considered.

Costs do not always come out as they have been budgeted. Sometimes this is because of problems well beyond the control of the manager. Other times, the manager should have the ability to control costs. Variance analysis is one aspect of cost accounting that has been receiving a growing amount of attention in hospitals as they attempt to control costs. As hospitals become more sophisticated in this area, there has been a growing shift toward flexible budgeting, a system that accounts for the portion of the variance from budget that is attributable to changes in volume and the associated change in variable costs.

Other Areas of Managerial Accounting. Besides including cost accounting, the general field of managerial accounting covers a wide variety of tools aimed at providing information to help the organization's managers to plan and control activities. These areas include financial information systems, ratio analysis, internal auditing, and budgeting.

Managerial accounting is concerned with the appropriate generation of financial information, the interpretation of information, and the accuracy of such information. Financial information systems are developed so that useful financial information can be generated on a timely basis. Ratio analysis is a technique for interpreting financial information and using it for improving management. Internal audits are useful for verifying the accuracy of the organization's financial information. Budgeting allows the organization to gain the advantages of working from a plan rather than on an ad hoc basis.

The generation of financial information is a critical need, and one that is the responsibility of all managers. Information must be both timely and useful. Many *financial information systems* gradually become outdated. Often one result of this process is that an overburdened financial information system is incapable of generating new, valuable reports because of the efforts going into generating reports that no one is any longer using. All managers must take the responsibility for seeing to the discontinuance of such reports and must demand the generation of reports that would provide useful information. With the great changes imposed by DRGs the type of information of interest to managers is changing dramatically. New types of information must be generated for an organization to remain competitive.

A ratio is simply one number compared to another; *ratio analysis* is a technique of managerial accounting that uses information available from financial accounting reports and the financial information system to compare numbers and develop relationships that can be useful for managers. For example, inventory turnover compares inventory used to inventory on hand. If it is determined that the inventory turnover is much slower than that of other hospitals, this may indicate inefficiency in the organization and use of inventory. It might be possible to lower the inventory levels. That would allow for spending less on inventory each year, thereby becoming more profitable. Such ratio analysis is commonly performed by financial officers. However, it is likely that ratio analysis could be used fruitfully by a wide variety of managers by determining relationships that provide useful information, and then obtaining the financial information to calculate those ratios and track those relationships over time.

Neither financial information nor ratios will be of much use unless the information is accurate. *Internal auditing* is a function of managerial accounting aimed at ensuring that the organization's financial records are accurate and that the assets of the organization are safeguarded. Human beings are a necessary part of all accounting systems. Human beings, however, are error-prone and subject to temptation. The accounting systems of an organization are designed to have checks and controls that automatically uncover most errors and that make frauds and embezzlements difficult. Nevertheless, errors and embezzlements do occur. The internal audit process is one in which the organization reviews its financial information to ensure that the system is functioning correctly, minimizing errors and preventing embezzlement. That an internal auditing process exists and may well discover theft is in fact one of the biggest preventives to theft.

Another managerial accounting focus is in the area of *budgeting*. Of particular budgeting interest for managerial accounting are the long-range budget, the program budget, and the operating budget. The capital budget and cash budget are other crucial aspects of the budgeting process; they are discussed later in the "Finance" section of this chapter.

The *long-range budget* attempts to plan the organization's direction for several years into the future. Without long-range planning, organizations tend to drift, with each year being largely a repetition of the previous year. It is easy to continue doing what has been done. It is much harder to make significant changes. The long-range planning process forces managers to set goals for where the organization should be in five years. That process allows for recognition of desired growth and change. It also forces the organization to make a commitment to move toward those goals.

Programming is the process of deciding on the major changes in the programs offered by the organization. It is the programming process that helps the organization to move from where it is today to where the long-range plan has indicated it wants to be in five years. Techniques such as *planning, programming budget systems* (PPBS) and *zero-base budgeting* (ZBB) help managers in this planning effort. The process of developing budgets for new programs or changes in existing programs is a difficult one, not only spanning time but cutting across many different departments as well.

The *operating budget* focuses on the revenues and expenses for the coming year. However, such a process has many complex elements, including appropriate forecasting of workloads, staffing, supplies, and expenses. It also requires the integration of the major programming changes coming out of the long-range plan and the programming process. The budgeting process should ideally be a rational one, with adjustments to the budget being based on issues such as patient acuity and on the least costly ways to provide care. Financial aspects of the budget must be integrated into patient acuity systems and staffing requirements. Arbitrary budget cuts fail to use the budget's information content as to what we get for our money spent in each department of the institution.

Managerial accounting provides information in many additional areas not discussed here. The key to managerial accounting is that it supplies any financial information that could be useful for decision making.

Finance

The last of the three areas of financial management, finance, deals with the financial resources of the organization. Safeguarding the financial solvency of the organization and ensuring the accomplishment of the financial goals of the organization are the key goals of finance. Finance accomplishes these goals by careful management of the sources and uses of the organization's financial resources.

Where does cash come from and how is it spent? On the surface, an easy issue: Cash comes from patients and is spent to provide them with services. In reality, a very complex issue. Rates must be established and reimbursement rules followed. Capital assets must be paid for long before patient revenues are received. Inventory levels, receivables, and payables must be carefully managed to avoid unnecessarily high interest costs. Cash inflows and outflows must be carefully timed. A working relationship with banks must be developed.

To a great extent, the information needed to make effective managerial decisions in these areas may be thought of as falling within the general definition of managerial accounting. In some areas, the distinction between managerial accounting and managerial finance is often vague. This is not surprising; managerial accountants claim as their territory the provision of financial information for planning and control. Certainly information about the organization's sources and uses of cash falls within that broad rubric. On the other hand, treasurers, guarding the financial resources of the organization, extend their domain from cash and investments to receivables and inventory.

Thus, management of inventory and other short-term resources, cash budgeting, and decisions regarding capital expenditures are topics claimed by both disciplines. But managerial accounting provides an exclusive focus on cost accounting, while finance claims an exclusive focus on sources of long-term financing, leasing, and banking relationships. The overlap between managerial accounting and finance is usually not a major issue with either controllers or treasurers, both reporting to a chief financial officer who determines the allocation of responsibilities.

Many techniques of financial management exist to help in handling the variety of problems concerning financial resources, whether they are exclusively finance issues or areas that overlap extensively with managerial accounting. For example, *working capital management* is a subfield of both finance and managerial accounting that focuses on the management of short-term assets and short-term liabilities. How soon should we pay our suppliers for items we have purchased? Not too soon, because payment requires us to take our money out of an interest-bearing bank account. The sooner we pay, the less interest we earn. On the other hand, not too late, or our suppliers will surely refuse to continue supplying us with their products.

How much cash should be kept in the bank for emergencies? Not too much, because money in the bank could be invested in new technology to expand the services offered by the hospital. But not too little, or we might run short on cash to meet our payroll. That could have a costly negative impact on morale.

How much inventory should we keep on hand? Inventory does not earn interest the way money in a bank does. Nor does it provide the services to our community that new technology could offer. On the other hand, we cannot afford to run out of a critical supply item.

As one can quickly see, in the area of working capital management the financial manager walks a tightrope. The desired goal is one of neither too much nor too little. However, a number of techniques exist to help in this process. Inventory can be ordered based on mathematical *economic order quantity* calculations. Cash balances can be monitored by the Baumol or Miller *cash optimization* formulas.

Once we determine when to pay, we must manage the resources in a way that allows us to operationalize the decision. For example, if we have cash that will be needed in several weeks or months to pay for some obligation, we cannot use that cash for a capital acquisition or we will be unable to make the upcoming payment. In that case we must find the best short-term investment to optimize the interim earnings of that money. On the other hand, we must know when sufficient cash will be on hand to make capital acquisitions.

The key is to have a projection of when cash is expected to be received and when cash will have to be paid. Such a projection can allow for carefully planned borrowing or investing. It can allow determination of when cash will be available for capital acquisitions. This projection takes the form of a *cash budget*.

Although cash budgeting is rarely the nurses' domain, it is clearly of interest to nurse managers. Suppose that a capital item is found to be profitable. We should go out and buy it. Yet the financial officers are not always so agreeable. Why? The mere fact that some investment is profitable does not mean that the organization has enough cash to undertake the acquisition.

Budgeting the cash flow of a hospital or other health organization is a complex process. Even though a capital item is profitable over its multiyear lifetime, we will undoubtedly have to pay more cash *now* to acquire it than we will receive this year because of it. The promise of ultimate profits does not solve the current problem of where to get the cash to pay for it. This type of problem is compounded by issues such as the seasonality of patient flow. Patient load may be heavy in the winter, creating large payrolls and outlays for supplies accompanied by high heating costs. Yet we may not receive payment from those patients until the spring, when occupancy is low.

The ability to budget cash flows depends in great part on revenues. This turns our focus to the process of setting hospital charges, forecasting patient volumes, and budgeting for revenues. Rate setting is a complex process that concerns adding a markup to our costs, the same as any business would. However, for health care organizations we have the added problems of complying with the complex rules for governmental and insurance company reimbursement, treatment of indigent patients, and the need to earn profits for expansion and for the latest technology. We also face the problem of pricing our services in a competitive marketplace.

In addition, long-term assets and long-term liabilities generate substantial problems for financial officers to deal with. Should we buy a piece of equipment or lease it? Should we borrow major amounts of cash from a bank, or should we issue a bond? Do we have the financial standing for a bond issuance to be feasible? If so, is our financial standing good enough for us to seek a bond rating? If interest rates fall substantially, should we refinance our outstanding debt? How do we maintain excellent bank relations so that we can borrow quickly at a reasonable rate?

Again, there are techniques of financial management that aid in handling these questions. Should we buy equipment or lease it? This question requires an understanding of the qualitative benefits of ownership weighed against the flexibility of a lease. However, it also requires an analysis of the amount of money spent and when it is spent. That analysis is based on a financial management technique known as present-value methodology, which is part of the larger process of capital budgeting.

Capital budgets are needed because some expenditures provide benefits for a number of years. To assess the cost of such items relative to the current year's revenues would be unfairly harsh. It might never seem to be financially feasible to acquire some essential piece of equipment. However, when such items are separated out of the operating budget, it becomes possible to understand their costs, relative to the benefits they provide over a period of years.

A problem arises because we have to pay for capital items at the time they are acquired, even though they are used over a period of years. The lag in use of the equipment and building also creates a lag in the receipt of revenues. In a tight financial environment this creates a critical problem because there is a distinct relationship between time and money. Money today is more valuable than money in the future.

To prove this to yourself, just consider whether you have a preference for receiving your paycheck this month or two years from now. Do you mind waiting two years for pay for work done last month? Of course, because you need the money now. Certainly, you could borrow the money you need now and repay the bank in two years, but you would have to pay interest.

The same is true for organizations. If we buy equipment today and pay for it today, there is a cost related to having to wait for several years to get the money back. There is at least the cost of the interest we pay a bank if we borrowed the money. Capital budgeting has a tool referred to as *present-value* or *discounted cash flow methodology,* which allows us to make the appropriate calculations so that our capital item decisions can consider the impact of the time value of money.

Thus we can compare the initial outlay related to buying an asset to the payments on a lease that are spread out over time. Using present value methods we can supplement qualitative analysis with an understanding of the complex financial implications of capital expenditure alternatives.

Once a decision is made to make a capital expenditure there is the question of where the money will come from to pay for it. Perhaps the money will be available from revenues from past patients. Often, however, it is necessary to borrow a substantial portion of the money needed. Should we borrow from a bank or issue a bond to raise money? Banks are more convenient, quicker, and have much lower costs related to the borrowing transaction. Bonds are extremely costly to issue, involving many lawyers, bond underwriters, advisers, and so on. However, bonds also tend to carry a lower interest rate than bank loans.

If the amount of money involved is great enough, the lower interest rate will justify the higher costs related to the initial issuance of the bond. Typically this requires the amount borrowed to be very large, and bond issuances occur only for major capital projects. A number of years will likely go by between bond issuances. Their rarity makes the process one of the most difficult tasks faced by financial managers.

The task is compounded by the fact that we cannot issue a bond unless we clearly have the capacity to repay the money we borrow through the bond issuance. Financial feasibility studies must be undertaken to evaluate whether we do in fact have that capacity. Furthermore, the financial strength of our organization must be evaluated. If we can obtain a good bond rating from an independent rating agency — Standard and Poor's or Moody's — we can lower our bond cost. That is because these agencies tell the public through their ratings how risky our organization is. The more risky, the higher the interest rate lenders demand.

Alternatively, we can arrange for a bond issuance to be insured by one of the associations of insurance companies— MBIA or AMBAC—that insure bondholders against failure to pay interest or principal. However, the insurance is expensive and is only worthwhile if it will likely lower the interest rate we have to pay by enough to offset the cost of the insurance.

Although bond issuances have a major impact on health care organizations, for the most part they are rare events reserved for major expansions or replacements of facilities. On a more routine basis financial managers focus on the management of existing resources in such a way as to keep the organization financially safe and to allow the organization to maximize the services that can be offered, given the resources available.

Summary

Financial management is an area of growing concern for nurses in management positions. Yet nurse managers for the most part are faced with the obstacle of coming into contact with specific elements of the financial "trees" without ever gaining a perspective on the financial "forest." The goal of this chapter was to step back from many of the day-to-day specifics of financial management with which nurse managers must deal. Instead, the framework that the specific techniques and details fit into has been examined, with the hope of providing an overview of the goals, aspirations, and techniques of financial management.

References

Bolandis, J. L. *Hospital Finance: A Comprehensive Case Approach.* Rockville, Md.: Aspen, 1982.

Broyles, R. W. *Hospital Accounting Practice.* Vol. II. Rockville, Md.: Aspen, 1982.

Cleverly, W. O. (ed.). *Handbook of Health Care Accounting and Finance.* Rockville, Md.: Aspen, 1982.

Davidson, S., Stickneyk, C. P., and Weil, R. L. *Financial Accounting: An Introduction to Concepts, Methods, and Uses.* (4th ed.) Chicago: Dryden Press, 1985.

Dermer, J. *Management Planning and Control Systems.* Homewood, Ill.: Irwin, 1977.

Dillon, Ray D. *Zero-Base Budgeting for Health Care Institutions.* Rockville, Md.: Aspen, 1979.

Dominiak, G. F., and Louderback, J. G. *Managerial Accounting.* (4th ed.) Boston: Kent, 1985.

Finkler, S. A. *The Complete Guide to Finance and Accounting for Nonfinancial Managers.* Englewood Cliffs, N.J.: Prentice-Hall, 1983.

Finkler, S. A. *Budgeting Concepts for Nurse Managers.* Orlando, Fla.: Grune and Stratton, 1984.

Finkler, S. A. (ed.). *Hospital Cost Accounting Advisor.* Rockville, Md.: Aspen, published monthly.

Frank, C. W. *Maximizing Hospital Cash Resources.* Rockville, Md.: Aspen, 1978.

Healthcare Financial Management. Chicago: Healthcare Financial Management Association, published monthly.

Herkimer, A. G. *Understanding Hospital Financial Management.* (2nd ed.) Rockville, Md.: Aspen, 1986.

Horngren, C. T. *Introduction to Financial Accounting.* (2nd ed.) Englewood Cliffs, N.J.: Prentice-Hall, 1984.

Killough, L. N., and Leininger, W. E. *Cost Accounting: Concepts and Techniques for Management.* St. Paul, Minn.: West, 1984.

Louderback, J. G., and Dominiak, G. F. *Managerial Accounting.* (2nd ed.) Belmont, Calif.: Wadsworth, 1978.

Modern Healthcare. Chicago: Crain Communications, published biweekly.

Rowland, H. S., and Rowland, B. L. *Hospital Administration Handbook.* Rockville, Md.: Aspen, 1984.

CHAPTER 6

Operations Research as a Strategic Management Tool

John C. Hershey

What is health care management? The *Report of the Commission on Education for Health Administration* (1975, p. 15) defined it as "planning, organizing, directing, controlling, and coordinating the resources and procedures by which needs and demands for health and medical care and a healthful environment are fulfilled by the provision of specific services to individual clients, organizations, and communities." Rakich, Longest, and Darr (1985, pp. 6–7) define it as "the process, composed of the set of inter-related social and technical functions and activities, occurring within a formal organizational setting for the purpose of accomplishing predetermined objectives through utilization of human and other resources." Others have similar definitions, typically emphasizing the activities of planning, design, implementation, coordination, evaluation, and control. But a common thread in any discussion of these management activities, after definitions are given, is the emphasis on the importance of good *decision making*. The quality of decisions determines the success, or even survival, of organizations.

Management draws on many disciplines — organizational behavior, operations research, financial management, marketing, accounting, and so forth. This chapter focuses on one of these disciplines — operations research — and its role in the health care management decision process. (Other terms that can roughly be used as synonyms for operations research are *management science, quantitative business analysis, operations analysis, operations management, operations engineering,* and *industrial engineering*

The operations research approach is based on the conviction that, to cope with the vast complexity of today's health care system, managers need to think about decisions in a systematic and scientific, rather than a disjointed and purely intuitive, manner. This is done by constructing quantitative models that typically focus on a part of the vast complexity of the real world. These models provide a simple, efficient representation of the overall decision problem. Because they consider only part of the problem, the recommendations from such models should typically *not* be used as a complete basis for action. Nevertheless, they can serve as important aids in the decision process. Models can help the manager see the problem more clearly, offer possible solutions that otherwise might not be found, and even redirect management's intuition. When it is most successful, operations research offers *qualitative* insight from *quantitative* analysis.

Before proceeding to a more complete description of operations research and its application to health care management, consider the following case example. (This case was written by the author for the Johnson & Johnson–Wharton Fellows Program. The microcomputer program developed for this case, described later in this chapter, was written with the assistance of Stephanie Barrett and Michael Chang.)

General Hospital Outpatient Clinic

You are an associate administrator at General Hospital, a 500-bed facility in a metropolitan area of approximately 2 million people. General Hospital currently operates a small outpatient clinic where, at present, three physicians are scheduled to see patients from 8:00 A.M. to 5:00 P.M. weekdays.

The past few days have been filled with meetings that have not exactly done wonders for your self-image. Morale among the professional and administrative staffs at the clinic is at an all-time low. The physicians are complaining that, too often, they are "wasting their time" in the clinic because they are idle.

They claim that on some days they have up to two hours of idle time.

At the same time there have been a growing number of patient complaints that they must wait for up to three hours or more to see a physician. The administrators scheduling the patients blame the problem on no-shows and walk-in patients (those without appointments). The physicians blame the problem on the administrators. Most importantly, the chief of operations blames you, since the clinic has been under your administration for the past three years.

Clinic Operations. Patients fall into two categories: those with appointments and walk-ins. Most types of patients are assigned to specific physicians. Patients with appointments have priority; walk-ins must wait until their physician is free.

Appointments are made in fifteen-minute blocks, starting at 8:00 A.M. There are also five scheduled breaks throughout the day, of varying lengths of time. There are a total of twenty-five appointment blocks potentially available, as shown in Table 6.1.

The receptionist will make appointments for a physician up to the approved load, which is currently 84 percent. At this level, twenty-one appointments are made for each physician, leaving four vacant appointment blocks. These are scattered throughout the day, at different times for different physicians, to balance out the office load.

Currently, the physicians arrive promptly at 8:15 A.M. and are available to begin seeing patients. Breaks are delayed if the physician is seeing a patient or if a patient scheduled for an appointment block before the break is still waiting to be seen. Once physicians start a break, they are not available for service until the scheduled duration of the break is complete.

In addition to their clinic responsibilities the physicians are periodically called away from the clinic to attend to emergency cases elsewhere in the hospital. These calls are out of the control of clinic administration. Each physician averages about 1.5 emergency calls per day, each lasting an average of thirty minutes, although actual amounts vary by physician and by day.

Table 6.1. Appointment Blocks at
General Hospital Outpatient Clinic.

8:00	Block	1	12:30		BREAK
8:15	Block	2	12:45		BREAK
8:30	Block	3	1:00	Block	13
8:45	Block	4	1:15	Block	14
9:00	BREAK		1:30	Block	15
9:15	Block	5	1:45	Block	16
9:30	Block	6	2:00	Block	17
9:45	Block	7	2:15		BREAK
10:00	BREAK		2:30		BREAK
10:15	BREAK		2:45	Block	18
10:30	Block	8	3:00	Block	19
10:45	Block	9	3:15	Block	20
11:00	Block	10	3:30	Block	21
11:15	Block	11	3:45		BREAK
11:30	Block	12	4:00	Block	22
11:45	BREAK		4:15	Block	23
12:00	BREAK		4:30	Block	24
12:15	BREAK		4:45	Block	25

On the average, patients with appointments arrive at the clinic ten minutes early, although specific patients may arrive as much as thirty-five minutes early or fifteen minutes late. An average of 10 percent of patients with scheduled appointments fail to show up at all. Patients check in with the receptionist on arrival and wait for their physician to become free.

There are an average of six walk-in patients per day at the clinic, although this varies from day to day. These patients are assigned a physician on checking in with the receptionist and must wait for that physician to become free.

Patients come to the clinic for a variety of ailments. The specific complaint is recorded in the medical records, but no formal classification system is in use. Each patient is with a physician for an average of fourteen minutes, ranging from six to twenty-four minutes for an individual patient.

Policy Alternatives. After giving the problem a great deal of thought, you have come up with four possible changes in the current clinic procedures that you think might help alleviate some of the perceived problems:

1. Change the current load factor (percentage of available appointments filled). Increasing the load factor will improve the utilization of physician time but will create longer patient waits. Decreasing the load factor will have the opposite effect.

2. Encourage the physicians to arrive at the clinic either earlier or later. Currently, they arrive at 8:15 A.M. because they like to build up a "cushion" at the beginning of the day to take care of late patient arrivals or patient no-shows. If the physicians arrived promptly at 8:00 A.M., there would be some reduction in patient waiting time at the expense of even greater physician idle time. If the physicians arrived later, at 8:30 A.M., for example, this would have the opposite effect.

3. The first two policy alternatives represent changes that would address one of your problems (physician idle time or patient waiting time) but would exacerbate your other problem. Each of the next two alternatives is an idea that might simultaneously help with both problems. One idea is to mount a campaign to decrease the number of patient no-shows. For example, you might hire additional part-time help at the clinic to call and remind each scheduled patient when she or he is due to be seen. If you could cut no-shows, you could simultaneously cut the current load factor enough to produce the same "effective" load that you currently have. The advantage would be that the additional open appointment slots could be distributed evenly over the day rather than occurring at random owing to the unpredictability of no-shows.

4. Finally, you are considering whether it might be possible to increase patient punctuality. At present, scheduled patients arrive as much as thirty-five minutes early or fifteen minutes late. It would seem that more punctuality could decrease both patient waiting and physician idle time. You are not quite sure how you could influence patients to be more prompt, but before attempting anything you wonder how much it would help to solve your problems.

These all seem like reasonable ideas, but your immediate question is what to do next. You have discussed these policy changes with the physicians and the administrative staff, but they are concerned about the costs and are skeptical about the benefits. What you would really like is some way to predict the effects of the policy changes, one at a time and in combination, on the relationship between patient waiting time and physician idle time. Perhaps a model would help to make these predictions. It might even suggest other policy changes you have not yet considered. If a model is developed, you feel it should be flexible enough to adapt to future changes in the outpatient clinic, such as its size, days, and hours of operation, and patient characteristics.

What Is Operations Research?

This case description is an example of a health care management problem that can benefit from operations research. We will return to General Hospital. First, however, I will describe the operations research approach and discuss the role of management in successful applications.

Operations research is a scientific approach to improving the quality of management decisions in situations in which there is considerable complexity and uncertainty. It is a primarily *quantitative* approach that involves defining, analyzing, and solving decision problems using mathematical models. These models use numbers, symbols, equalities, and inequalities to represent the logic, information, and interrelations inherent in the management problems, and they tend to use decision criteria that can be *objectively measured.*

The methods of operations research are drawn from many disciplines, including mathematics, economics, statistics, computer science, and organizational behavior. In the 1940s and 1950s most operations researchers were people whose primary education and experience had been in one of these disciplines. Today it is still important for an individual entering this field to have sound training in the basic methodologies of these areas. But it is also now common for these professionals to take their specialized academic training in a formal academic program leading to a degree in operations research (or "management science" or any of the other labels given in the introduction to this chapter). It is also common for operations researchers with complementary skills to work together as teams on large, complicated problems.

The breadth of applications is very wide. Operations research is used in industry, health care institutions, the military, government agencies, transportation, and so forth—essentially anywhere where there are complex problems of management planning, coordination, and control. What is common in all these applications is the construction and solution of models that attempt to abstract the essence of certain management problems.

The stages in conducting an operations research study can be described as follows:

1. Formulating the problem
2. Constructing a mathematical model to represent the system under study
3. Deriving a solution from the model
4. Testing the model and the solution derived from it
5. Establishing controls over the solution
6. Putting the solution to work: implementation

These stages are discussed in detail in Hillier and Lieberman (1986, pp. 16–25).

In the first stage—developing a well-defined statement of the problem—it is important to observe carefully the system whose behavior must be understood and explained. This includes defining the appropriate objectives, the constraints on what is possible, and the potential alternative courses of action. This phase of an operations research study must be conducted with considerable care and should be continually reexamined as the study proceeds, to avoid wasted effort later looking for the best solution to the wrong problem. Drucker (1974, pp. 466–470) describes the tendency of the Japanese to emphasize the importance of *defining the question* when making management decisions, as opposed to the Western emphasis on *finding the answer*. He argues that greater attention to problem definition can often lead to more effective decision making.

As part of the first stage, the operations researcher will define two types of variables: *controllable* variables (decision variables that are under the control of the decision maker) and *uncontrollable* variables (numerical descriptions of conditions in the environment that restrict the latitude of the decision maker). In the course of constructing a model, mathematical formulas are devised to represent the interrelationships among these controllable and uncontrollable variables. The next stage is to calculate a mathematical solution. The solution indicates what action or actions best meet the objectives of the decision maker, *according to the model.*

Models can be classified as *optimization* models or *simulation* models. Most applications use optimization models — that is, they are designed to give the optimal or best solution directly. For example, this may involve finding values for the decision variables that optimize one of the objectives and give satisfactory levels of performance on the other objectives. (Many nurse staffing models take this approach.) The techniques used in optimization models include linear programming, nonlinear programming, inventory theory, project scheduling, and decision analysis. Another approach is to "experiment" with the model by "simulating" the results that would occur with different decisions. (Simulation models are commonly used for studying health facility scheduling problems, such as those presented in the General Hospital example.) Simulation models differ from optimization models in two ways. First, they are not designed to find the optimal solution directly but instead allow the decision maker to experiment with a number of proposed solutions and then reach conclusions on the basis of a comparison of the results. Second, simulation models generally focus on operations in great detail. The system is studied as it operates over time, and the effects of one time period's results on the next are included in the model. Among the many books describing the mathematical techniques of operations research are Baker and Kropp (1984), Hillier and Lieberman (1986), and Wagner (1969).

The recommendations from an operations research model can only be as good as the assumptions that were made when it was formulated. The model is an idealized representation of reality, but it may still be a good enough approximation. Clever methods can be devised to test the model by use of historical data or data from another organizational setting. In addition, it is usually important to establish systematic information-collection procedures to ensure that the anticipated changes in performance actually take place. Often the operations researcher can recommend adjustments in the solution that take into account ongoing, unanticipated changes in the system.

As described by Hillier and Lieberman (1986, p. 24), the implementation stage involves two steps. First, the operations researcher gives management a careful explanation of the solution to be adopted and how it relates to the realities of the operational setting. Second, these two parties share the responsibility for developing procedures to put the solution into operation. Of course, the operations researcher must monitor the initial experience with the decision chosen and must recommend any necessary modifications.

The Role of Management

Operations research supports real-world decision making by helping the manager visualize problems more clearly, clarifying his or her objectives, and suggesting possible solutions. To be successful, the recommendations of any modeling effort not only must be technically valid but also must be organizationally realistic. If this is to be accomplished, management must be closely involved in all stages of the analysis.

The operations researcher's forte is mathematical analysis. But the manager best understands the organizational setting. Management has a critical role to play in ensuring that the correct problem is being addressed, that the qualifying assumptions in the model are realistic, and that the formulation of the problem is appropriate. There is an inevitable trade-off that must be made between a model's tractability and its realism, a trade-off that is "too important to be left to the analyst." The model should predict outcomes reasonably well and be consistent with organizational reality.

Inevitably, the model will be an abstraction of those factors that are considered most relevant to the problem, and there will be qualitative factors that are not a formal part of the model. The manager must use some intuition and common sense to find an appropriate balance between quantitative and qualitative factors.

Management is best able to evaluate the impact of proposed solutions on the organization, particularly if these solutions require people to change behavior or if they are threatening to anyone's interests. New incentives or organizational processes may be required to get the solutions accepted. Perhaps the best way to ensure implementation success is to have all affected parties participate, to some degree, in developing the model.

Finally, the manager should be aware of a very powerful capability inherent in any operations research model: the ability to identify how the recommendations depend on each of the assumptions of the model. This capability is called *sensitivity analysis*. Sensitivity analysis can inform management as to how the optimal solution is expected to change as a function of changes in the value of any specific uncontrollable variable, or changes in the model formulation. For example, management might learn that the solution is relatively insensitive to changes in the assumed values for some uncontrollable variables, and thus need not be overly concerned about possible error in estimating these values. On the other hand, the solution may be quite sensitive to changes in some of the other assumed values, suggesting that it might be wise to give these values extra attention or even to commission a statistical forecasting study to predict them more precisely.

It has been said that once the optimal decision has been found, the analysis has just begun. This emphasizes the importance of challenging the underlying assumptions of any model by asking a number of "what if" questions. What if demand declines? What if costs increase? What if the patient mix changes? By exploring the answers to these questions, the manager not only can learn about the sensitivity of decisions to underlying assumptions but in the process can gain a better intuitive understanding of the operating environment.

General Hospital Outpatient Clinic Revisited:
An Operations Research Approach

In General Hospital there are two perceived problems: excess physician idle time and excess patient waiting time. For purposes of analysis, the four policy alternatives presented in the case — load factor, physician arrival time, patient no-shows, and patient punctuality — can serve as the controllable variables. Other variables, such as clinic hours, service times, scheduling policies, and specialization of tasks, can be taken as uncontrollable variables for the initial analysis. Of course, these designations of controllable and uncontrollable variables may change over time.

An outpatient simulation model has been developed to give insight into the operations of the General Hospital Outpatient Clinic. The model simulates the actual operation of the clinic for fifteen days, keeping track of patient arrivals, schedules, service times, scheduled breaks, emergencies, the number of patients in the waiting room, physician utilization, and the length of the workday. The computer program gives a number of summary statistics after the simulation is complete. These summary statistics provide information on physician utilization, patient waiting time, and other measures of clinic operations.

When one runs the program, one can change any or all of the four decision variables corresponding to the four policy alternatives. If none are changed, they are kept at their current values, which correspond to the current clinic operations. The four decision variables, along with their current values (in parentheses), are as follows:

1. Patient load (84 percent)
2. Physicians' arrival time (fifteen minutes late)
3. Patient no-show probability (10 percent)
4. Latest arrival time for a patient with an appointment (currently set at fifteen minutes late: Because the average arrival time is always ten minutes early and the model assumes a symmetric probability distribution, a change in latest arrival time automatically produces an equal and opposite change in earliest arrival time)

Table 6.2 shows the form of the output provided by the program. This table corresponds to the current system (base case). It also provides a brief description of each line of output.

One way to analyze the four policy alternatives is to make changes one at a time, holding the other three constant at their current levels. For example, the load factor might be varied from as low as 60 percent to as high as 100 percent, or the physicians might arrive as early as 8:00 A.M. or as late as 8:30 A.M. Essentially, these are experiments that use the model to explore alternative policies and their interactions and to see how they affect different measures of physician idle time and patient waiting time. Of course, one can also carry out sensitivity analysis by changing assumptions or the values of uncontrollable variables and then rerunning the experiments.

Experience with this particular simulation model shows that the load factor has a marked effect on both physician utilization measures and patient waiting-time measures. What is more surprising is that, for any given load factor, patient no-shows and patient punctuality have an imperceptible effect on these measures. There is little to be gained from attempting these changes. On the other hand, having the physicians arrive earlier yields great reductions in patient waiting time with a very modest increase in physician idle time. For example, with the base case, by having physicians arrive at 8:00 A.M., forty-six minutes of walk-in-patient waiting time is saved for each minute of increased physician idle time.

After changes are implemented, the administrator must carefully monitor the actual performance measures and compare them with those predicted by the model. The model might well evolve over time as the administrator gains experience with trying out different policies, thinks of new policies to be tested, and challenges some of the underlying assumptions.

Operations Research in the Service Sector

Many applications of operations research have taken place in goods-producing organizations. Specific examples include manufacturing strategy, production policy, inventory control, scheduling

Table 6.2. Results of Fifteen-Day Simulation of the Base Case for General Hospital Outpatient Clinic.

CURRENT SIMULATION PARAMETER SETTINGS:
1. Doctor load factor: .84
2. Doctor arrival time: 15.00
3. Probability of patient no-show: .10
4. Latest arrival time for an appointment: 15.00

Summary Statistics — Run 15

	Doctor 1 Mean	Min/Max	Doctor 2 Mean	Min/Max	Doctor 3 Mean	Min/Max	Aggregate Mean	Min/Max	
NO-SHOWS	1.60	0. 4.	2.33	0. 5.	2.07	0. 5.	2.00	0. 5.	Avg. no. of no-shows per day
EMERGENCIES	1.13	0. 3.	1.20	0. 3.	1.47	0. 4.	1.27	0. 4.	Avg. no. of emergency breaks per day
WALK-INS	2.13	0. 5.	1.53	0. 3.	2.20	0. 6.	1.96	0. 6.	Avg. no. of walk-ins per day
PATIENT COUNT	21.53	19. 25.	20.20	18. 23.	21.13	16. 26.	20.96	16. 26.	Avg. total patient count per day (appts. + walk-ins – no-shows)
DOCTORS' HOURS	8.94	8.7 9.5	8.95	8.7 9.4	9.06	8.7 10.7	8.98	8.7 10.7	Avg. time from arrival to departure
TOTAL SERVICE TIME	336.78	261. 393.	318.14	252. 389.	336.88	247. 475.	330.60	247. 475.	Avg. time with patients
TOTAL IDLE TIME	34.32	0. 113.	53.77	0. 108.	41.85	0. 111.	43.31	0. 113.	Avg. time idle
UTILIZATION	.907	.699 1.000	.855	.701 1.000	.885	.689 1.000	.882	.689 1.000	Service time/service time + idle time

	Average	Minimum	Maximum	No. of Observers
WAITING ROOM COUNT				
AVERAGE	4.33	1.	13.	822 – No. of patients in waiting room
WORST CASE	8.27	6.	13.	15 – Peak load in waiting room
WAIT TIMES				
PREAPPOINTMENT	10.29	– 13.93	34.90	855 – Waiting time before appt. for appointees
POSTAPPOINTMENT	11.29	– 30.00	105.83	855 – Waiting time from appt. to admission for appointees
APPOINTEES' TOTAL	21.58	.00	125.35	855 – Total waiting time for appointees
WALK-INS' TOTAL	113.21	.00	483.53	88 – Total waiting time for walk-ins
PERCENT WHO WAIT	87.07	63.16	93.65	15 – % of all patients who wait
HOURS OPEN	9.59	9.09	10.99	15 – Time from 8:00 to close of business

of personnel and facilities, facility location, production and distribution system, and quality control.

In part because of increased productivity in the manufacturing sector, the U.S. economy has shifted from one oriented primarily to goods manufacturing to one engaged primarily in the creation of service. Operations researchers are experiencing this same trend in their own employment opportunities. Their challenge is to enhance productivity in the service sector with the same success they have had in the manufacturing sector.

Operations research technology developed for goods-producing applications often cannot be transferred directly to service operations. Of course, some of the topics mentioned above, such as personnel scheduling and facility location, have relevance for service delivery. But their specific application to the service sector needs special attention. The provision of quality service as an objective, not a constraint, must be emphasized in service applications. Service, in turn, must be measured in terms of multiple criteria, and the affected parties will disagree on the relative importance of different criteria. The quantity of service is difficult to measure, and quality control is especially difficult to achieve. Service (usually) cannot be stored in inventory, awaiting a customer's order. Health care services, in particular, are crucially time dependent, are sometimes of an emergency nature, and cannot be deferred or "back-ordered" without incurring heavy penalties. Together, these last two points imply that demand variations usually must be absorbed through personnel allocations and reallocations rather than through inventory. Finally, because service is labor-intensive, the consequences of inefficient *personnel* organization, planning, and control need special attention.

Operations Research Applications in Health Care

Until recently, most applications of operations research in health care were in hospitals. During the past decade, however, an ever-growing number of studies have considered other aspects of health care delivery. These include planning and control in non-hospital delivery settings, regional planning, and medical decision making.

Reviews of the literature are given by Stimson and Stimson (1972) and Fries (1976, 1979, 1981). A collection of articles describing applications is provided by Boldy (1981). The main journals publishing health care operations research methods and applications are *Operations Research, Management Science, Health Services Research,* the *Journal of Medical Systems, Medical Care,* and *Medical Decision Making.*

One overriding feature of nearly all health operations research studies is the necessity to measure health quality or health status. Typically, a measure or index is developed as a surrogate for health status. The index can be used to provide some indication of before-and-after effects of interventions or as a measure that is to be maximized in an operations research optimization model. A review of health status measures is given by Warner and Luce (1982).

Within hospitals, the main target for study has been nurse staffing and scheduling. Because of the importance of this topic and its particular relevance for this book, nurse staffing systems will be described in detail in the next section of this chapter. Other hospital applications have included process design and facility planning, admission scheduling, inventory control and materials management, and sizing and scheduling of special facilities. In addition, many of the utilization review and quality insurance systems used in hospitals are based in large measure on operations research models.

In nonhospital settings, operations research has been used for facility location, personnel planning and the effects of personnel substitution, appointment systems, determining ambulance requirements and deployment, and regional blood banking. Regional health planning models (starting with the Hill-Burton formula, possibly the first operations research "model") have become increasingly sophisticated (Cohen and Hershey, 1980).

Finally, perhaps the fastest-growing application area is clinical decision making. An analysis technique called *decision analysis* is now taught in medical schools, and it has had a substantial impact on health screening decisions, the analysis of management alternatives for specific patients, and the choice of diagnostic tests. An excellent overview of this field is given in Weinstein and others (1980). *Medical Decision Making* is the primary journal in this field, although other journals, such as the *New England Journal of Medicine,* publish articles on clinical decision making.

Nurse Staffing Management

Since nursing service is the largest single cost center in the hospital, and since hospitals are under increasing pressure to bring about improved cost control, it is understandable that hospital managers have turned to operations researchers to find more efficient ways of organizing nursing resources. In this section, those elements of the nurse staffing process that are worthy of investigation will be identified and managers will be directed toward more comprehensive and fruitful problem-solving approaches. The suggestions are presented in the context of a conceptual framework that contains all the interrelated management tasks that directly affect nursing staff utilization and performance. Some of the material in this section is abstracted from Wandel and Hershey (1975).

Tactical Nurse Staffing Decisions. The nurse staffing process can be conceptualized as a hierarchy of three tactical decision levels, which will be called corrective allocations, shift scheduling, and personnel planning.

Within a shift, the staff capacities among units may be adjusted by using float, part-time, relief, pulling, overtime, and voluntary absenteeism. (*Float* refers to a pool of cross-trained nurses who are floated among units to smooth demand fluctuations; *pulling* refers to the temporary reallocation of a nurse to a unit other than the one in which he or she normally works.) These *corrective allocations* should be based on the individual's preferences and capabilities, and they are restricted by shift schedules and the employees' capabilities.

The second decision level is *shift scheduling*—that is, uniform and smooth matching between expected workload and staff capacity among units on a week-to-week and day-to-day basis. For each employee, days on and off, as well as shift rotation and time for classes, are determined. The individual's preferences and talents should be considered to bring about high personnel satisfaction and to ensure that personal capabilities are made use of in the best way.

These two "scheduling" levels concern the utilization of personnel already existing within the organization; they have a known mix of specialization and experience. However, the long-term balance of numbers and capability of nursing personnel among units is obtained by hiring, training, transferring between jobs, and discharging. This decision level can be called *personnel planning*. Because of the time lags involved, personnel planning actions should be taken early to meet anticipated long-term fluctuations in demand and supply.

Interdependence of the Tactical Decisions. The interdependence of these three levels is often neglected. Each level is constrained by available resources, by previous commitments made at higher levels, and by the degree of flexibility for later correction at lower levels. Therefore, each decision level is strongly dependent on the other two; one level should not be considered in isolation.

The week-to-week shift scheduling decisions and the shift-by-shift corrective allocations obviously depend on the numbers and capabilities of personnel established through the personnel planning process. On the other hand, the range and flexibility of shift scheduling and corrective allocation options available to management should be known so that their performance can be anticipated and included in the staffing decisions of the personnel planning process. Thus, the overall staff requirements cannot be fully assessed until it has been decided how fluctuations in load are to be accommodated. If overtime, for example, provides the only flexibility in short-term scheduling, the full-time staff requirements might be substantially higher than if part-time help were also available.

Furthermore, decisions at each level should be coordinated with future and past events within the level itself. Coordination with the future should be accomplished through the planning stages: forecasting, tentative planning, action planning, and execution. All the uncontrollable variables that have a major influence on the staffing process should be forecast. Examples of these variables are workloads for each skill category, hiring prospects, turnover, and absenteeism. However, the planning process at each level should also be dependent on the other two. The plans can be said to be "gliding" or "rolling"; that is, an action plan for one level should be the basis for a tentative plan for the level below, and they should be updated and made firmer as execution is approached and more information becomes available.

Performance Monitoring, Strategic Decisions, and Coordination with Other Hospital Activities. The three tactical decision levels are depicted in Figure 6.1. It can be seen from this figure that there are important interactions between these tactical nurse staffing decision levels and other management activities. As shown in the box at the left in Figure 6.1, coordination with the past should be accomplished through a *performance monitoring* system, which should (1) take the inventory (numbers and capabilities) of employed personnel; (2) measure, control, evaluate, and correct staffing performance; and (3) gather statistics to be used as a basis for forecasting.

There are also important *strategic policy and design decisions* in a hospital that restrict the number of alternatives available at each of the three tactical decision levels. This aspect is depicted in the box at the top in Figure 6.1. Examples include policies about the use of float personnel, the control of admissions, the skill mix of the nursing personnel, and the number of nurses in the training pool at any point in time. These policies should be part of any investigation into new methods to improve productivity.

Finally, it is important to consider the interdependence between nurse staffing and *other hospital activities,* shown at the right in Figure 6.1. Each nurse staffing level should cooperate with equivalent and related levels in the demand and facility control systems. That is, corrective allocation should be coordinated with task assignment; shift scheduling with the scheduling of admissions, operating rooms, and treatment and supportive services; and personnel planning with budgeting, recruitment, training, and facility planning.

Figure 6.1. The Nurse Staffing System.

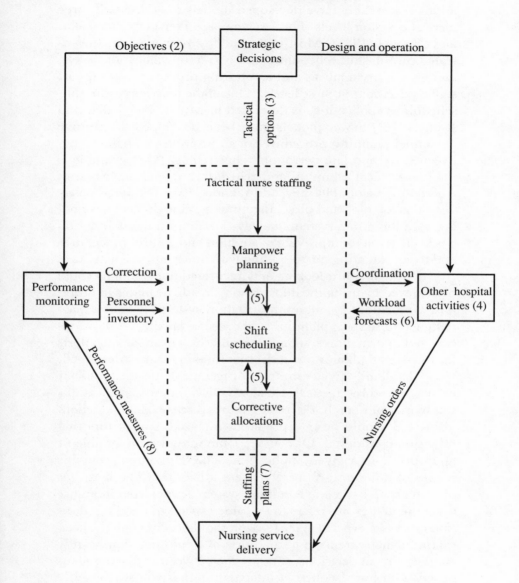

Note: Numbers in parentheses refer to row numbers in Table 6.3.

Technical Specifications for a Nurse Staffing System. Operations researchers have developed models to address all three
tactical decision levels. For a review, see Hershey, Pierskalla,
and Wandel (1981). Most nurse staffing research has concen-
trated on the shift scheduling and corrective allocation levels,
and on activity analysis and forecasting procedures to support
staffing decisions at these levels. (One of the most successful shift
scheduling applications is described in Miller, Pierskalla, and
Rath, 1976.) Fewer models have been developed to improve
personnel planning procedures or to improve the balance between early and late personnel adjustments. (One example is
the hierarchical planning and scheduling model described in
Abernathy, Baloff, Hershey, and Wandel, 1973.) Strategic policy
decisions to guide and direct the nurse staffing process have not
been explored in a systematic way. Finally, minimal attention
has been given to improving evaluation and control procedures
and to coordinating nurse staffing with other hospital activities.

More forward-looking and integrated nurse staffing could
be achieved by using the information already available in hospitals. Unfortunately, many information systems have not been
designed to support planning and decision making. A decision-
oriented information system that could support modeling efforts
for nurse staff planning and decision making is now described.

Table 6.3 gives examples of technical specifications for
each of the three tactical decision levels. These specifications
summarize most of the desirable features discussed in this section.
Table 6.3 should be interpreted as a checklist of factors that
might be considered. Of course, some may not be feasible or
appropriate in a given application. The left column contains
names of different groups of system attributes. The locations
of each group in the nurse staffing system are depicted in Figure
6.1. The first group refers to the time aspects of the three decision processes, where (1) the horizon should be far enough ahead
that a further extension of the horizon would not significantly
change current decisions; (2) the time between reviewing plans
depends on how frequently information that will significantly
change the plans becomes available; and (3) the planning period
is the smallest interval during which the decision variables can
be considered constant.

The objectives and tactical options for each decision level are listed in rows 2 and 3. Row 4 indicates the other hospital activities with which each level should be coordinated, and the information needed for coordination among the tactical decision levels is shown in row 5.

Row 6 lists variables for which probability distribution should be forecasted. Most of them are uncontrollable, but some control can be achieved by influencing the processes that give rise to the uncertainties. The integrative factors (rows 4 and 5) have this purpose.

The multitude of possible nurse staffing decisions precludes an exhaustive evaluation of all alternatives even if all pertinent information were available. Therefore, it would be desirable to have decision models built into the information system that synthesize the available information into plans. Row 7 gives examples of such plans that might be used as the basis for the manager's staffing actions.

Before actions are taken, the manager could perform sensitivity analyses. That is, the models could be used to analyze "what if" questions, such as: What will happen to costs if demand is redistributed in time or among units through admission control? What will be the effect of changing certain policy constraints on costs? What would be the value of having better forecasts? Such analysis may result in changes in strategic decisions, collection of more information, or negotiations with other functional areas in the hospital.

The performance of a nurse staffing system is dependent not only on the planning process but also on the evaluation and control process. The outcomes of both controllable actions and uncontrollable events should be measured frequently. Outcomes such as those shown in row 8 can be compared with forecasts, decisions, previous outcomes, and other standards, and differences can be analyzed. The purpose of such performance analysis would be to (1) augment the manager's understanding of the process, (2) assign responsibility, (3) revise plans and schedules, and (4) improve future decisions by suggesting better procedures or policies. As in the planning process, quantitative models might be of value to reduce and analyze data, to infer causes of differences, and to analyze "what-would-have-happened-if" types of questions.

Table 6.3. Example Specifications for a Nurse Staffing System.

		Tactical Decision Levels		
	Mobility Planning	*Shift Scheduling*	*Corrective Allocations*	
(1) Horizon/review/period	Year/month/month	Month/week/shift	Day/shift/two hours	
(2) Objectives (expectations and standards)	Low cost High personnel satisfaction High flexibility High service level	Equitable and high workload/staff ratios among units Equitable and high schedule satisfaction among personnel High substitutability	Smooth workload/staff ratios Continuity of care High quality of care Low cost Equitable and high personnel satisfaction	
Relative priorities are controllable				
(3) Tactical options	Recruitment Promotion Transfer Training Vacation Departure	Shift rotation Pattern of days on Stretch of days on Individual constraints Minimal coverage Skill mix	Float Pulling Part-time Relief Overtime Voluntary absenteeism	
Controllable in the long run				
(4) Other hospital activities (external coordination)	Budgeting Capacity planning Training programming Recruitment programming Admission control	Admission control Care planning Facility scheduling Support-service planning Training scheduling	Patient reallocation Treatment scheduling Task specification Task assignment	
Controllable through negotiations				
(5) Information for internal coordination	Personnel inventory Individual preferences Planned reallocations Scheduling flexibility	Available personnel Preferences Capabilities Planned absenteeism Allocation flexibility	Posted schedules Desires Substitutabilities Allocation commitments Productivity flexibility	
Partly controllable, partly past events				

(6) Forecasted (exogenous) variables	Admissions Patient mix Workload/patient and skill level Turnover Absenteeism Recruitment prospects	Workload/shift, unit, and skill level Absenteeism Substitutability	Nursing orders Emergency care needs Availability of part-time and relief Absenteeism Productivity
Uncontrollable future events	Salary Efficiency		
(7) Staffing plans (suggestions)	Aggregated manpower plans Individual development plans Recruitment programs Training programs Vacation schedules	Shift schedules Individual schedules Scheduled load/staff ratios Training schedules Admission suggestions	Daily reallocations Part-time, relief, and overtime schedules Decision rules for emergency corrections
Partly controllable future events	Target load/staff ratios Personnel cost budget		
(8) Performance measures	Workload/month, unit, and skill level Hours paid Hours worked Personnel cost Personnel inventory (number and skill) Turnover Personnel satisfaction Time to fill vacancies Reasons for departures	Workload/shift, unit, and skill level Hours available Hours training Absenteeism Hours rescheduled Schedule satisfaction Skill mix	Hours of care required, ordered, and given Quality of care process Patient satisfaction Hours of noncare Utilization of personnel Time to fill emergency care needs Personnel satisfaction
Controllable and uncontrollable past events			

Conclusions

Public regulations, new payment methods, and competitive forces will continue to increase the pressure on health institutions to contain costs. Operations research holds great promise for helping bring about improvements in productivity.

The techniques and models of operations research should be viewed as tools that help to augment, rather than replace, administrative judgment. Used properly, they can bring about new dimensions of problems, help clarify objectives, suggest options that might not be developed through intuition alone, and shed light on the implications of alternative actions.

References

Abernathy, W. J., Baloff, N., Hershey, J. C., and Wandel, S. E. "A Three-Stage Manpower Planning and Scheduling Model — A Service Sector Example." *Operations Research,* 1973, *21,* 693–711.

Baker, K. R., and Kropp, D. H. *Management Science.* New York: Wiley, 1984.

Boldy, D. (ed.). *Operational Research Applied to Health Services.* London: Croom Helm, 1981.

Cohen, M. A., and Hershey, J. C. *An Analysis of Regional Health Planning Methodologies.* Philadelphia: Leonard Davis Institute of Health Economics, University of Pennsylvania, 1980.

Drucker, P. F. *Management.* New York: Harper & Row, 1974.

Fries, B. E. "Bibliography of Operations Research in Health Care Systems." *Operations Research,* 1976, *25* (5), 801–820.

Fries, B. E. "Bibliography of Operations Research in Health Care Systems." *Operations Research,* 1979, *27* (2), 408–419.

Fries, B. E. "Applications of Operations Research to Health Care Delivery Systems." In D. A. B. Lindberg and P. L. Reichertz (eds.), *Lecture Notes in Medical Informatics.* Berlin: Springer-Verlag, 1981.

Hershey, J. C., Pierskalla, W., and Wandel, S. E. "Quantitative Methods for Nurse Staffing Management." In D. Boldy (ed.), *Operations Research Applied to Health Services.* London: Croom Helm, 1981.

Hillier, F. S., and Lieberman, G. J. *Introduction to Operations Research.* (4th ed.) Oakland, Calif.: Holden-Day, 1986.

Miller, H. E., Pierskalla, W. P., and Rath, G. J. "Nurse Scheduling Using Mathematical Programming." *Operations Research,* 1976, *24,* 856–870.

Rakich, J. S., Longest, B. B., and Darr, K. *Managing Health Services Organizations.* (2nd ed.) Philadelphia: Saunders, 1985.

Report of the Commission on Education for Health Administration. Vol. 1. Ann Arbor, Mich.: Health Administration Press, 1975.

Stimson, D. H., and Stimson, R. H. *Operations Research in Hospitals.* Chicago: Hospital Research and Educational Trust, 1972.

Wagner, H. M. *Principles of Operations Research.* Englewood Cliffs, N.J.: Prentice-Hall, 1969.

Wandel, S. E., and Hershey, J. C. "A Conceptual Framework for Nurse Staffing Management." *Omega,* 1975, *3,* 541–550.

Warner, K. E., and Luce, B. R. *Cost-Benefit and Cost-Effectiveness Analysis in Health Care.* Ann Arbor, Mich.: Health Administration Press, 1982.

Weinstein, M. C., and others. *Clinical Decision Analysis.* Philadelphia: Saunders, 1980.

CHAPTER 7

Assessing Electronic Tools and Information/Decision Support Systems

Cecile A. Feldman

Information technology is revolutionizing the way in which nurses assess, diagnose, plan, and deliver patient services. In a time of cost constraints, legal requirements, and quality concerns, computer capabilities are enabling care to be delivered in more economical and efficient ways. In addition, electronic tools are now a necessity in nursing management and administration. Computers give nurses the capability to store and quickly retrieve vast quantities of information. New systems guide nurses in interpreting information, managing operations, and researching future ones.

Today, nurse executives are being asked to make decisions regarding the design of hospital and nursing information systems, purchase of computer equipment, and use of computers in daily management activities. Given that the introduction of computer technology into the daily activities of nurse executives has been relatively recent, this chapter assumes that the reader has little if any experience with computers. The first part of the chapter describes how computers and electronic tools are used in nursing management. The second part describes the process involved in implementing an information system. The role of nurse managers in recommending, justifying, developing, managing, and utilizing information systems will also be discussed.

Nursing management information systems assist nurses in patient care, resource allocation, personnel management, policy planning, and decision making. Patient-care management systems retrieve, collect, store, transmit, and organize information about patient demographics, diagnoses, treatment plans, treatment interventions, and health outcomes. These information systems assist in patient care, patient education, quality monitoring, and nursing research. Resource allocation systems assist nurse managers in putting together nurses' schedules and quantify the demand for nursing care. Personnel management systems assist in maintaining individual nurse-employee data, including date of hire, work availability, performance capability, benefits, experience, education, length of service, salary, and educational development. Planning and policymaking systems include management information reports; nursing care costing systems, which report patient charges and revenues; and institutional financial management reports. Decision support systems provide programs that allow for investigation into the effects of management decisions. These support systems interface with operational databases and allow managers to make informed decisions quickly.

Electronic Tools

Computerized information systems consist of *hardware,* the physical components that comprise a computer system, and *software,* the set of instructions that control operations of the physical components of the computer.

There are four general categories of computer hardware: input devices, output devices, storage devices, and the computer's central processing unit. Input devices, such as keyboards, mice, touch screens, light pens, digitizers, and bar-code scanners, allow computer users to put information into the computer. Output devices, such as monitors and printers, allow users to retrieve information from the computer. Storage devices, such as magnetic tapes and disks, store information in an electronic format, and the central processing unit contains the silicon chips needed to process information. A more detailed overview of computer hardware can be found in Shelly and Cashman (1984).

Nursing departments utilize various types of electronic software tools including text processing, number crunching, database management, presentation, and communication systems.

General purpose off-the-shelf computer software gives nurse managers and their support staff tools to improve administrative and management activities. Over the past fifteen years text processors, number crunchers, database managers, presentation tools, and communication facilities have been developed and refined. These software packages, combined with the evolution of inexpensive desktop microcomputers, have brought these electronic tools into most offices.

Text Processing Tools. Document origination and refinement systems, *word processors,* have revolutionized secretarial responsibilities. At first glance it would seem that word processing would have little effect on nurse managers, but word processing is a powerful tool for increasing personal productivity. Nurse managers are constantly required to produce correspondence, reports, and protocol documents. Word processing tools eliminate the need to retype whole documents due to editorial or content changes. Letters and words can be inserted or deleted by a few keystrokes, and sections of text can easily be moved from one part of the document to another. Word processing allows for ongoing modification by eliminating the need to erase or retype entire segments of the document. Documents can be sorted electronically and later retrieved for modification. In addition, word processors can check documents for misspellings and grammatical errors, suggest alternative words (thesaurus capabilities), set margins and spacing, insert headers and footers, perform search-and-replace operations, and prepare outlines and/or tables of contents. Documents that can be prepared with a word processor include intraoffice memos, external correspondence, policy manuals, new program proposals, and patient-care plans.

How word processors are used within the nursing department will depend on personal work preferences. Currently there are three ways in which a nurse manager can use a word processor:

1.   The nurse manager prepares the document in longhand and a secretary or clerical staff member types the document into the word processing computer system.
2.   The nurse manager dictates the document and has the secretary transcribe the document by typing the document into the word processing system.
3.   The nurse manager generates the first draft of the document by typing the document directly into the word processing system.

In all cases refinements to the document are passed on to clerical personnel for entry into the computer. Many managers, executives, physicians, and nurses find that developing original documents on word processors results in considerable time saving. Many feel that first drafts tend to be better because changes are made when the initial document is drafted. Changes can easily be made, and confusing paper or dictation notes do not have to be interpreted by support personnel. Of course, use of a word processor is contingent on one's ability to type.

Number-Crunching Tools. *Electronic spreadsheets* are software programs that can remember a set of numbers and formulas. The computer performs calculations based on these numbers and formulas. The most powerful aspect of electronic spreadsheets is their ability to allow users to perform "what if" scenarios. The computer performs calculations based on assumptions that are operationalized by entering numbers and formulas. Any mathematical model that can be organized into a worksheet context, rows and columns, can be performed by an electronic spreadsheet.

A spreadsheet is made up of cells (see Figure 7.1). Each is labeled by the row and column in which the cell appears. Cells can contain text (labels), numbers, or formulas. Applications that should be put into electronic spreadsheets have the following characteristics: (1) many of the numbers are computational derivatives of other numbers in the worksheet, and (2) once prepared, if one or more numbers in the worksheet change, other numbers change accordingly. Like word processing documents,

Figure 7.1. Electronic Spreadsheets.

Cell A2 contains the text "Expenses."

Cell B3 contains the number "450,000."

	A	B	C	D	E
1		1990			
2	Expenses				
3	Personnel	450,000			
4	Benefits	90,000			
5	Supplies	150,000			
6	Travel	25,000			
7	Computer	10,000			
8	TOTAL	725,000			
9					
10					
11					
12					
13					
14					
15					

Cell B8 contains the formula "B3+B4+B5+B6+B7," which translates into 450,000+90,000+150,000+25,000+10,000, or 725,000.

Note: An electronic spreadsheet is made up of cells that contain text, numbers, or formulas.

spreadsheet templates and data can be electronically stored and retrieved for later use.

For example, the expense figures for a nursing department can be entered into the computer under the control of an electronic spreadsheet program. After the data have been entered and the total expense calculated, the CEO might ask how expenses would change if the occupancy rate increased by 7.5 percent. By entering the new occupancy rate, the nurse manager directs the spreadsheet to recalculate the expense values. Electronic spreadsheets are an invaluable tool for decision support. For nurse managers, electronic spreadsheets can be used to prepare budgets, performance reports, staffing schedules, patient acuity reports, quality assurance statistics, service utilization summaries, and cost allocation.

Normally, electronic spreadsheets are used in two different ways. If the manager is experienced in developing spreadsheets, then the manager can develop the spreadsheet without having to specify the model to auxiliary personnel. The manager performs "what if" scenarios interactively with the computer. However, if the manager is not experienced in spreadsheet usage, the nurse manager would have to describe to a programmer the data and calculations to be performed. The programmer would be responsible for developing the spreadsheet and then running the scenarios that the nurse manager specifies. The second option reduces the interactiveness potential of using a spreadsheet decision support model but still enables the nurse manager to take advantage of exploring the implications of various management decisions.

Statistical programs allow nurse managers to calculate frequencies, means, standard deviations, ranges, and various other statistical measures on employees, patients, occupying rates, discharge rates, length of stay, and other hospital data. For research and quality assurance programs, statistical tests can be performed on time-series or cross-sectional data. ANOVA, t test, chi square, and nonparametric statistics can easily be performed to compare groups of patients. Since it takes time to master statistical programs, nurse managers are likely to work closely with either a systems analyst or a statistician. Nurse managers would be given the computer output or document that summarizes the results of the statistical analysis.

Database Management. Database management software allows a collection of organized data to be retrieved in various formats. A computerized *database* is equivalent to a manual file system. A database consists of one or more *files.* Each file consists of *records.* Records consist of data items called *fields.* For example, a personnel file would contain a record for each employee for which information is being saved. A patient treatment file would contain a record for each patient, and an inventory file contains a record for each supply item. For the personnel file, potential data items consist of the employee's name, address, birth date, social security number, and home phone number (see Table 7.1). Data items in the inventory file include product name, vendor, name, unit cost, reorder quantity, and quantity on hand.

The database management software allows for the manager to manipulate data, arranging data in ascending or descending sequence and displaying all or selected data. Data are manipulated by specifying a few simple commands in English-like statements. The ability to retrieve information at electronic speeds is an important advantage to computerized databases. Sophisticated reports that require the selection of specific records, sorting of data, and combining of data from one file with data from another file can be generated. Database applications include equipment/supply inventory, staffing profiles, employee profiles, continuing education profiles, and CPR training monitoring.

Because database programs are still very complex and difficult to learn, most nurse managers requiring database applications will work closely with an information system programmer. The nurse manager is responsible for indicating what information (data items) is required and how the information is to be used. In addition, the nurse manager must design the reports that present the required information in a meaningful way. The programmer would be responsible for developing data-entry screens and the database reports. Normally, data-entry or clerical personnel would be responsible for entering information into the computerized database.

Table 7.1. Employee Personnel File.

	Data Item 1 Name	Data Item 2 Address	Data Item 3 Birth Date	Data Item 4 Social Security #	Data Item 4 Phone Number
Record 1	Ron Wong	100 First Street Philadelphia, PA 19104	October 1, 1955	111-11-1111	(215) 898-0001
Record 2	Maria Rodriguez	200 Second Street Philadelphia, PA 19104	November 15, 1952	222-22-2222	(215) 898-0002
Record 3	Jane Jones	300 Third Street Philadelphia, PA 19104	April 20, 1962	333-33-3333	(215) 898-0003

Note: A personnel file consists of records. The file contains one record for each employee. Each employee record contains data items such as employee's name, address, birth date, social security number, and phone number.

Presentation Tools. To senior-level executives presenting new programs, making recommendations to change existing programs, and being responsible for making periodic reports on departmental activities, the availability of tools to quickly and inexpensively generate professional-looking documents, graphs, slides, and overheads is essential. The recent introduction of desktop microcomputers, which have graphic capabilities, has moved these activities from the institution's graphic artist office onto the nursing department secretary's desk.

Charting programs enable a series of numbers to be turned into graphs, which provide easy interpretation. Current technology allows the use of color, which can call attention to numbers of particular interest. Graphs can be produced in a matter of seconds in contrast to waiting days or weeks for a graphic artist to draw each graph by hand.

Laser Printers. In conjunction with *desktop publishing,* software permits clerical workers to generate reports that appear to have been professionally designed and typeset. Desktop publishing programs enable a clerical worker to combine text, graphics, and drawings all in one document. They give the clerical worker greater control over spacing and page layouts. Master pages allow the user to design a universal layout pattern, including elements such as page numbers and headers that can be placed on both left- and right-hand pages. If the nursing department wishes to produce newsletters or brochures, secretaries can produce the documents, saving the nursing department much time and expense by eliminating the need to use a graphic artist and printer.

Desktop Presentation. Software assists users in organizing presentation notes and producing overhead or 35mm slides. Most presentation software consists of an outliner and 35mm slide generator. The outliner assists the presenter by providing a mechanism for organizing notes for a presentation. Notes can also be entered into the computer, and a printout of the slides, outline, and notes can be generated for use at the presentation. Graphs or drawings from other computer software programs can be combined with the outline material to produce slide images. The slide generator converts the slide images into either overhead or 35mm slides. Because the multitudes of colors, print fonts, and slide formats make it very difficult for nonartists to design presentations that are attractive and effective, most programs come with predefined templates, designed by professional artists. These templates suggest color combinations, print styles, and font sizes that have proven to be esthetically pleasing and effective. Presentation programs also have slide sorters, which enable presenters to rearrange their slides as if they were using a light box.

Because these programs tend to be difficult to learn, a clerical or support staff member would develop the slides or overheads under the direction of the nurse manager. If the hospital owns a film recorder, a device that can record the electronic images produced by the presentation software onto film, slides can be generated in less than twenty-four hours. (If Polaroid 35mm film is used, the film can be developed in less than five minutes.) If your hospital does not own a film recorder, the electronic slides can be electronically mailed to a slide service, which transfers the slide images to film and develops the film. These service bureaus return developed slides within forty-eight to seventy-two hours. Overheads can be produced in a matter of minutes, since laser printers and plotters can be used to print overhead transparency film.

As with desktop publishing, desktop presentation can save the nursing department time and money by obviating the need to have graphic artists develop, design, and produce slides and overheads for presentations.

Communication Utilities. Advances in communication technologies permit users to communicate with other managers via *electronic mail*. In order to use electronic mail facilities your personal computers must be joined together via cable so that one person's computer can communicate with other computers. Messages, in the form of letters or memorandums, can be sent to others in the network. The messages are stored on a centrally located computer until the receiving user is ready to read his or her mail. When reading electronic mail, the user has the option to print messages and/or make appropriate responses by returning a message electronically. Electronic mail reduces the amount of paper correspondence. It permits messages to be sent faster and eliminates the need for having a staff member hand-deliver correspondence or risk sending memoranda through interoffice mail.

Personal computer networks connect individual personal computers so as to create a workgroup of personnel computers. A *local-area network* covers a limited geographic area. Local-area networks allow for hardware resource sharing, information resource sharing, and electronic mail and text transfer. The sharing of peripheral hardware devices minimizes the cost of computerization by reducing the number and size of peripheral devices needed. For example, one laser printer, which costs from $1,500 to $5,500, can be shared by a number of personal computers, eliminating the need to buy a separate printer for each computer workstation. Information sharing allows anyone on the local-area network to share documents stored by others on the local-area network. Thus if you drafted a document and saved the document on the local-area-network *file saver,* your secretary would have immediate access to the document, allowing for immediate changes and updates without having to keep track of *floppy disks*.

Information/Decision Support Systems

Over the past few years computer applications that support clinical, management, and administrative responsibilities have grown exponentially. As senior management one of your responsibilities is to identify activities and functions that can be more efficiently performed with information technology. Recommendations as to what resources are needed to satisfy these needs must be documented and justified.

Types of Information/Decision Support Systems. Most hospital data are captured and stored by *electronic data processing systems*. An electronic data processing (EDP) system performs transaction processing functions, which include admissions, billing, discharges, accounts payable, and payroll. Transaction processing focuses on data collection, data storage, data processing, and data reporting. EDP systems are detail oriented and monitor daily operations.

A management information system is a computer-based system able to integrate data from various sources to provide the information necessary for middle management (Hicks, 1984). It is oriented toward operations management. The systems summarize information collected by EDP systems and utilize reports that are produced on a periodic basis, usually weekly or monthly, as opposed to the EDP system's daily reports. Good *management information systems* (MIS) have the capability of integrating and summarizing data collected by different EDP systems to produce relevant management information. An integral part of the MIS is a *database management system* (DBMS), which aids in the management and manipulation of EDP data. Examples of reports produced by a hospital MIS include monthly income and expense reports, monthly staff workload analysis, and monthly occupancy, length of stay, and acuity rates. As management decisions are made, effects of these decisions will appear on reports produced by the MIS. For example, if the administration decides that staffing must decrease by 5 percent to improve profitability, changes in the hospital's income and expense reports and staffing reports would be apparent.

Management information systems also consist of *decision support systems* (DSS). These are "an integrated set of computer tools that allow a decision maker to interact directly with computers to retrieve information useful in making semistructured and unstructured decisions" (Hicks, 1984, p. 404). A DSS is more than just a set of computer software tools. These systems are decision focused and are aimed at top-level managers and executive decision makers. The systems are designed to support personal decision-making styles of individual executives and are user initiated and controlled. Emphasis is on flexibility, adaptability, and immediate response. DSS allow managers to play "what if" scenarios, incremental assumptions, and risk and other forms of analysis. Examples of DSS that might be used in a hospital setting include profitability projections and staff workload projections. Figure 7.2 summarizes the three types of

Figure 7.2. Hierarchy of Information Systems.

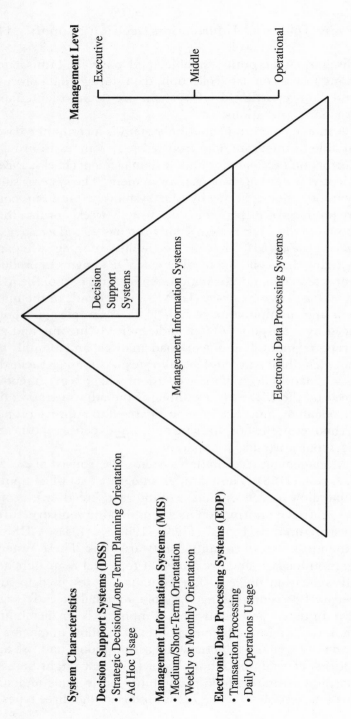

Management Level

Executive

Middle

Operational

Decision Support Systems

Management Information Systems

Electronic Data Processing Systems

System Characteristics

Decision Support Systems (DSS)
• Strategic Decision/Long-Term Planning Orientation
• Ad Hoc Usage

Management Information Systems (MIS)
• Medium/Short-Term Orientation
• Weekly or Monthly Orientation

Electronic Data Processing Systems (EDP)
• Transaction Processing
• Daily Operations Usage

Note: Hospital information systems consist of electronic data processing systems (EDP), management information systems (MIS), and decision support systems (DSS).

information systems (EDP, MIS, and DSS) that are commonly found in a hospital environment.

A decision support system is built on a database, a simulation model, and a user interface by which managers or appropriate support staff can interact. It is the simulation model that allows the DSS to be used for top-level decision making. By mathematically modeling the operations of a hospital, the impact of potential decisions can be tested. Executive-level managers are not involved in the actual building of the DSS. Rather, the manager specifies the decision for which a DSS could be helpful and defines the appropriate model that is needed. A DSS builder who is familiar with the problem and also with information system technology assembles the necessary resources to implement the DSS. An information system technical support person develops the additional information system capabilities needed, such as new databases, new models, additional data displays, and interaction formats. The manager could interact directly with the DSS, interact with the DSS through an intermediary such as a clerical assistant who can help in pushing the buttons at the terminal, or interact through a higher-level staff assistant, who interacts with the system by making suggestions as to what actions can be taken.

System Justification, Design, and Implementation. When it is believed that electronic tools — EDP, MIS, or DSS — can improve the efficiency and effectiveness of the nursing service/hospital's operations, a process that starts with a needs analysis and ends with new system implementation and evaluation is initiated (see Figure 7.3). The *needs analysis* begins the system specification process and serves as a basis on which hospital management will approve or disapprove the project. Once the needs analysis is completed, a *request for proposal* (RFP) must be written. The RFP details the required system capabilities. System vendors respond to the RFP by submitting a proposal detailing how their system meets or can be modified to meet the hospital's needs. Based on the proposals a vendor is selected or a decision is made to develop custom software. Implementation of the system includes detailed system specifications, coding (if the

**Figure 7.3. Overview of Information System
Justification, Design, and Implementation Process.**

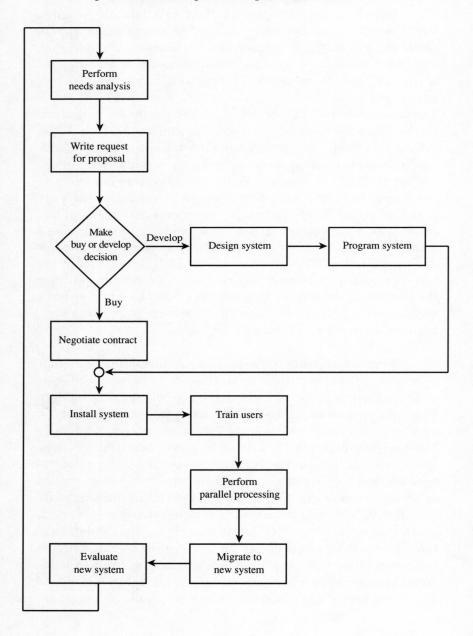

system is to be custom developed), operationalizing the system, training users in the operations of the system, and evaluation of the system to see whether or not it is meeting its original goals and objectives.

The Needs Analysis. In determining potential activities or functions that can benefit by computerization, one should exhaust all potential sources for ideas. As a minimum, it would be helpful to consult staff nurses, nurse managers, and peers at other hospitals.

Staff nurses and nurse managers will be best able to point out areas of potential increase in productivity by computerization. Involved with day-to-day patient care and operational activities, they are the individuals who will use this technology, and they therefore must be a part of the needs assessment and implementation process.

It is very useful to make site visits to peer institutions that are known to have good computer systems. Site visits often reveal innovative systems that have been overlooked. Reviewing the past experiences of peer institutions can often save months of investigative time and can provide a basis by which common pitfalls can be avoided. Not only should you be concentrating on the system (that is, computer screens and reports), but it is extremely important that you carefully examine the hospital's management structure and protocols. If your hospital is radically different from the one you are site visiting, it is highly unlikely that a system that works well at the peer institution will work at your hospital. It is important to remember that computer systems do not perform clinical care or administrative functions. Computers are only tools that make nurse performance more efficient.

Once specific areas that can benefit from computerization have been identified, a formal *needs assessment* document should be prepared. The needs analysis documents the information needs of the nursing service. Included in the analysis is a description of the present information system, specifications of current and future information needs, and an analysis of the current system's ability to accommodate current and future needs. In defining the present system it is important to determine exactly how the current system operates and the extent to which it services current information needs. Conditions that limit the existing system's ability to meet new needs must be identified. Potential limitations include application software limitations (software customized to perform specific nursing/hospital tasks), operating system limitations (software such as programming languages, file structures, and computer operating systems), and computer hardware limitations. In addition, the process, personnel, data collected, facilities, and costs associated with operating the existing system must be identified.

In the description of future information needs of the nursing service/hospital, resource and technical constraints must be kept in mind. Federal, state, and local regulations must be considered. It is imperative that information needed to make informed strategic and tactical decisions — not just information required for daily operations and reporting purposes — be included.

The final part of the needs analysis requires comparing current with future resources and needs. If no differences exist, or if these differences are modest, it is highly probable that a new system is not needed. If the differences are modest, it is highly probable that changes can be made to the existing system, again eliminating the need to buy or create a new one. If there is no current system, or if substantial differences exist, the hospital most likely requires a new system. At this point, an analysis that compares the costs of acquiring and implementing the new system versus the benefits the hospital anticipates receiving from the new system must be made (Drazen, 1983; Schmitz, 1987).

Potential benefits include increased timeliness, accuracy, completeness, and easier accessibility to information used in patient care. Potential costs include the monetary cost of obtaining and implementing the information system and increased labor costs. It should be remembered that some of the most important benefits, such as improved quality of patient care, can be extremely difficult if not impossible to quantify. It is only worthwhile acquiring and implementing a new system if the value of the new system is greater than the cost of developing/implementing the new system.

The needs assessment document serves three purposes. First, the document outlines the nursing department's goals, how computers can help the department better meet these goals, what resources are needed, and what options are available for implementing systems to satisfy these needs. Second, the document serves as a basis on which your hospital's administration can evaluate your needs. It is your best attempt at justifying why resources should be directed at the nursing department. The needs assessment document should justify your needs and present a convincing argument for computerization. Third, the document will help in your initial selection of potential hardware, software, and consultant service vendors. Vendors will be able to gain an understanding of what your needs and desires are.

In addition to describing activities that would benefit by computerization, the needs assessment document should indicate hospital-specific characteristics that will help in determining machine capacity and system complexity. These indicators include number of beds, staff size, yearly admissions, average length of stay, and other indicators important to activities requiring computerization.

Anticipated personnel savings and/or new required personnel should be indicated. In most cases, computerization will not eliminate the need for people. Rather, staff nurses will be freed from performing clerical tasks and thus be able to perform more patient-care activities. Additional clerical staff with special data-entry skills will probably be required. Special requirements such as data security, system failure backup systems, and data archive systems should also be included.

Request for Proposal. Once senior management has agreed that an information system is needed, a request for proposal, which details specific requirements for both hardware and software, must be established. The RFP serves as a communication tool between buyer and seller. It documents the hospital's needs and is used to select vendors. The RFP is an opportunity for the hospital to document systematically its needs, independent of which system vendors can supply. Technological, functional, and economic issues are addressed in the RFP. The RFP should include (Hicks, 1984):

1.   A description of the proposed application(s). If possible, the data to be maintained, screens needed, reports desired, and the overall system flow are to be included. This description should be as detailed as possible. Stating that a system must contain a registration system is not detailed enough.

2.   System reliability requirements. System reliability requirements include whether or not the system must be functional twenty-four hours per day and how critical it is to have a backup system that is immediately operational should the primary system fail.

3.   Backup requirements. These include the electronic medium onto which data are to be archived and battery backup requirements for power failures.

4.   Vendor service requirements.

5.   List of specific hardware or software features required, including special printer speed or disk capacity requirements. For example, if computers are to be used in patient education programs, it is necessary to have special hardware (that is, videodisc technology, touch screens, or voice recognition hardware) to make patient use of the computer as easy and effective as possible. Another example would be that if terminals were to be placed at every bedside, the main computer system must be able to accommodate a large number of concurrent transactions.

6.   Criteria for evaluating proposals.

7.   Plans for vendor demonstrations of hardware and software.

8.   Implementation schedule.

9.   Price constraints.

10. Specific questions about characteristics of the vendor's hardware and software.

11. Procedures for clarifying and submitting the RFP. The individual to contact for RFP clarification and the scheduled date for submitting the proposal should be included.

12. Information about the vendor. This includes their business plans, size of the company, other projects of similar scope, and financial statements. Vendors should also be asked to supply the names and phone numbers of individuals at other hospitals as references.

Once proposals from potential vendors have been received, a process that results in vendor selection must be initiated. If possible, it is helpful to develop an objective scoring mechanism. A scoring mechanism for which each requirement is ranked on a scale from 1 to 3 (1 = requirement not met, 2 = requirement partially met, 3 = requirement fully met) allows a "total" score to be calculated for each vendor. Those vendors with top scores can be called in for presentations. During the presentation vendors are required to explain their system or consulting services. Questions can be asked to clarify uncertainties. Vendor responses to questions will help in evaluating the vendor's ability to meet the hospital's requirements.

When evaluating the proposals received from vendors, it is extremely beneficial to visit peer hospitals utilizing the proposed systems. Site visits should be performed without the sales representative, because existing clients will be more honest if a vendor representative is not present. During a site visit evaluations can be made regarding user interaction with the system, since it will be possible to observe the system in operation. Evaluations can also be made regarding screen format. It is important to assess the impact of the system on the personnel using it. The system's ease of use should be determined. Analysis should focus on the proposed system's ability to help your staff perform their jobs in a more efficient and effective manner.

Topics for discussion include the following questions:

1. Was the system delivered and installed on schedule?
2. Was the vendor open to modifications?
3. Does the vendor supply adequate support?
4. Were your expectations met?
5. Was the vendor's price quotation accurate or were there additional hidden costs?
6. What is the opinion of "users" of the installed system?

Sometimes desired systems are so new that no proven installations exist. In this case you will have to weigh the risk of choosing new technology with unproven application programs against the risks of choosing an existing system with proven functionality but that might not cope with your rapidly changing information needs (Schmitz, 1987).

Before the final vendor can be selected the vendor's financial and management stability must be determined. Since computer systems have a life span of five to ten years, your confidence in the vendor's ability and commitment to support the product for several years is important. Financial data can be obtained from the company's audited financial statements. It is often useful to look at the company's strategic and/or long-range plan. A meeting with the company's vice president or president can also assist in determining a company's commitment to the hospital and/or nursing information system. Do not rely on the marketing claims or the sales representative's word.

The proposals should not be evaluated on the basis of price alone. Cost is not always related to the functionality of the system. When looking at the economics of the proposal, one must compare the cost of collected data with the value of the information. It is often difficult to make this judgment because a prospective cost-benefit analysis must be performed. Hospitals tend to overestimate benefits and underestimate costs. Computer salespeople often deemphasize costs and stress benefits. It is therefore necessary to perform a realistic cost-benefit study to the widest extent possible. Only after objectively evaluating the proposals, meeting with the companies' technical personnel, talking to current and past clients, determining the vendor's future commitment to their product, and determining the real cost can one make an informed decision.

Because information systems tend to be extremely costly, it is important that all the people who participated in developing the needs analysis and request for proposal be included in the final decision-making stage. Involving a large number of people will ensure commitment to the project.

Be careful not to be convinced that your needs are not what you originally indicated. Some system vendors will try to convince you that your hospital really needs the capabilities of the system that they are proposing rather than the needs defined in your needs analysis. This often occurs when suppliers are unable to provide the functions that were originally specified. Keep in mind that a fine line exists between the system supplier who recommends changes to improve your proposed system in good faith and the system supplier who is attempting to change a user's mind simply to make a sale (Schmitz, 1987).

Negotiations and Contracts. If a decision is made to buy existing hardware and/or software, a negotiation process to result in a contract agreeable to both sides must be initiated. As a general rule, vendors will ask the hospital to sign a form contract. These contracts put together by the vendor have been designed to minimize vendor risks and maximize vendor profits. Thus the hospital should insist that a mutually beneficial contract be negotiated, one which protects both system vendor and hospital.

Both hospital and system vendor must be willing to negotiate and strike a fair balance. A successful relationship is one in which the contract is rarely if ever consulted. Each should try to understand the other's situation. Sales representatives often overstate a system's potential in their enthusiasm for making a sale. On the other hand, hospitals often withhold important information because they do not feel it is important. Therefore the RFP serves as an important document on which contract negotiations can be based (Entin, 1982; Schmitz, 1987). Both the system vendor and the hospital must realize that the system will be successful if by selling the system the vendor gains benefit and the system meets the hospital's needs. Successful implementation only results if the hospital works with the system vendor and the hospital is involved in the entire implementation process. For example, the hospital should take on some of the responsibilities of system testing, training personnel, developing procedures, and scheduling installation/implementation activities.

It is important that an attorney familiar with software licensing agreements be consulted. In contract negotiations, delivery schedules, fee schedules, system acceptance, performance criteria, warranties, rights to programs, equipment liability, acts of God, maintenance of equipment, operation of the software and equipment, software support, user physical facilities, default actions, arbitration, and other factors must be included (Entin, 1982; Schmitz, 1987). Establishing a contract forces the hospital to consider what issues are important in installation and operation of the system. The contract binds the vendor to deliver specific goods and services to the hospital in a designated time frame. It also binds the hospital to certain levels of performance, such as providing environmental controls for computer hardware and providing the data and personnel needed for adequately testing the new sytem.

Delivery dates for hardware, software, and documentation should be clearly written out because perceptions of conditions, attitudes, and relationships between hospital and system supplier can change. Fees are obviously a very important part of the contract. Both parties must agree on the fees for hardware, software, installation training, and consulting, and on the schedule of payments for ongoing support and maintenance of the system over a specified period of time. In addition, exactly what is included in the system support and maintenance should be made clear.

Normally a vendor will require full payment when the hardware/software is delivered. This means that the hospital is required to pay long before the product has been proven to operate as promised. It is therefore desirable to condition payments on completion of acceptance testing. If the project is lengthy, periodic payments should be arranged with payments skewed toward the end of the project.

Be careful when a system vendor says that all upgrades to the system are included in the yearly support and maintenance. Software vendors have a tradition of calling upgrades new products, which would then obligate you to buy new products at retail price. Agreements should be negotiated where for a specified period of time support and maintenance fees include both upgrades and new products. In addition maximum increases (either as an absolute amount or as a factor tied to an economic indicator such as the CPI) for software support and maintenance for at least a five- to ten-year period should be included. Since hospitals incur sizable initial licensing fees, training costs, and system validation costs, it is highly unlikely that a hospital will quickly migrate to another software system. Software vendors often take advantage of this by charging retail fees for support and maintenance after the initial contract runs out.

If appropriate, the contract should specify that charges do not include federal, state, or local taxes. Since many hospitals are not-for-profit, this must be communicated to the system vendor so that buying/selling transactions take the hospital's tax-exempt status into account.

It is advisable to state in the contract the conditions under which the user accepts the system and payments are made. Speed, reliability, and performance-testing criteria to be used to measure the system's acceptability are to be specified. That time should not exceed three seconds is an example of measurable and objective criteria. As mentioned earlier, these criteria should have been included in the RFP.

Warranties and maintenance agreements usually require the hospital to provide a suitable environment for the hardware. It is generally the user's responsibility to prepare the site for the hardware. Site preparation includes renovations to provide for appropriate security and access to the computer CPU and hardware peripherals, such as tape drives, disk packs, and printers. In addition, electrical and environmental conditions (humidity and temperature) must be met.

Arrival of hardware must be timed after necessary renovations are completed. In user areas, the locations of terminals with proper electrical supplies and lighting must be provided.

Most system vendors provide a ninety-day or one-year warranty on the hardware components. Thus the contract must specify the agreed-on long-term maintenance conditions and costs of the maintenance agreement. Often standard maintenance agreements will only provide standard business hour maintenance service. This means that if a piece of equipment breaks at 9:00 P.M., a repair person will not be available to fix the problem until 9:00 A.M. the next day. Contracts can be negotiated for twenty-four-hour maintenance, but customers must be willing to incur additional costs. In addition, the contract should specify whether maintenance will be done on-site or whether the customer must provide for delivery of the defective hardware to the vendor. Arrangements in the contract should also be made for cases in which hardware must be removed for repairs or replacement. If hardware must be replaced, will the vendor supply another piece in its place until the replacement is received by the user organization and installed?

Who is responsible for equipment that is damaged by fire, water, or acts of God must also be specified. Some vendors will require the hospital to carry fire, earthquake, water, or other disaster insurance. If equipment is rented, the vendor will often assume liability for the equipment if there is no customer negligence. However, if equipment is owned by the customer, liability generally accrues to the user except in cases of negligence by the system vendor (Schmitz, 1987).

The contract always specifies the conditions under which the customer can use the software. In most cases, the hospital is buying a license that gives the hospital the right to use the software for a specific period of time. Since the hospital is not buying the software, the hospital does not own it and can therefore not resell the software to other health care organizations. The hospital cannot represent the software as being its own. In addition, system vendors will only provide support for the software if no changes are made to the system. If changes are made, the system vendor must be contracted to make the necessary changes. It is extremely unusual for a system vendor to support software that a hospital has modified.

The who, what, and how of hardware/software support should also be spelled out in the contract. Knowing the hours user support will be provided and how that support can be obtained is extremely important. For example, do you have twenty-four-hour access to an individual who can answer questions about the hardware/software? You should know whether or not the hardware/software support contact person(s) is (are) solely responsible for this software project, or if he or she is responsible for supporting many products. If the support person(s) is (are) responsible for many products, it is highly unlikely that he or she will be an expert on the hardware/software you have purchased. Agreement must be reached as to whether you will receive hardware/software support free, on a fixed monthly or yearly fee, or on a per-call or hourly basis.

Contracts usually specify conditions for which default is considered to have taken place. The default clause should specify the remedies available to both system vendor and hospital. For example, if a software vendor goes out of business, what rights does the hospital have to the software? Often provisions are written into the contract that require the software source code to be placed into escrow. If the software vendor goes out of business, the hospital has the right to obtain the source code and to use or modify it.

Implementation. If your hospital decides to custom develop an information system, systems personnel must be identified. Often programmers and system analysts from the hospital information system department will be assigned to the project. It is important that programmers and analysts be assigned to only one project at a time. If not, you will have little control over time schedules and priorities. The final detailed system design must be documented and agreed on. The detailed design translates the functional specification into a set of modules that can be implemented as computer programs. Executable code is then entered into the computer and debugged.

Although it might appear that custom-programming applications can be very time consuming, it should be understood that programming is usually only a small percentage of the total project's activities. As a rule of thumb, analysis and design represent 40 percent of a project's effort, coding of the application accounts for only 20 percent, and validation, training, and evaluation account for the last 40 percent (Blum and Orthner, 1986).

Trade-offs exist between customizing an application and its likelihood for successful implementation, timeliness, and user acceptance. Custom-built programs are customized to the user organization and thus are more likely to fit into the hospital's operations. However, custom programs are risky if there is poor project management. The possibility exists that you will end up with no executable code due to poor design or programming. In addition, it will take more time to implement a system that does not currently exist than a system that is "off the shelf."

When a program is being custom programmed, it is imperative that the system be developed and tested in small modules. Each program that is written must be individually tested and debugged. Module functions must be compared to the system specifications to ensure that all specifications have been met. Once the individual programs have been tested, they must be combined into modules, and each module must be independently tested. Finally, when all the modules have been tested, they must be combined and the system tested and compared against the initial requirements specification to see if the system has met the original system objectives.

Because most systems, both purchased and developed, operate in a changing environment, it is inevitable that changes will be required. If changes are not required, the system is not being utilized and most likely does not meet the users' needs. Requests for change is a sign that the system is being used. Normally more than half of the total lifetime cost for the system is for maintenance. Costs can run as high as 80 percent of the initial project costs (Blum and Orthner, 1986). Thus the ability to maintain the system should be considered as important as its initial acquisition/development. Maintenance can be divided into three types: (1) corrective maintenance — the identification and elimination of errors; (2) adaptive maintenance — the accommodation to changes in hardware, software, or other external forces; and (3) perfective maintenance — that is, the modification of the system to meet new or changed needs. On average, corrective maintenance often accounts for 20 percent of the maintenance effort, adaptive maintenance for 25 percent, and perfective maintenance for 55 percent (Blum and Orthner, 1986). After a while the costs and process of making changes to a system outweigh the costs of replacing the old system. Thus implementing a hospital information system cannot be looked at as a one-time expense/activity. Rather, information systems should be seen as an evolving entity that must continually change if they are to help an organization operate in a changing environment.

Whether you are implementing a "custom"-developed or "off-the-shelf" system, adequate training for system users must be provided. Users should be involved at the earliest point possible. As soon as system testing begins, users should be employed to evaluate the system. Users will provide the most realistic and accurate assessment of the system.

The training process can be broken down into two stages: (1) system orientation and (2) formal training. System orientation introduces the system to large groups of personnel. The purpose of the system and what benefits are to be realized along with required new work flow should be presented.

Formal training is provided to small groups of users. Information presented includes (1) computer terminology, (2) hardware operation demonstration, (3) descriptions of system functions, (4) demonstrations of each function, (5) delineation of policy and procedures, (6) manual backup system description, and (7) demonstration of printouts, reports, and labels.

Hands-on sessions in an informal environment are provided as part of the formal training. This part of the training process is the most important and most time consuming. Practical exercises that simulate the real environment must be developed. Interactive on-line teaching programs (tutorials) or one-on-one training with the actual system in use are potential hands-on training modalities. On-line interactive teaching programs guide the future user through each function with questions and prompts. They allow for future users to progress at their own pace and review specific functions without having to involve training personnel. The weakness of this training program is that tutorials do not convey all the nuances and more advanced capabilities of the system. The advantages of this method of training include low cost, because minimal training personnel are required, and flexible training time (users can use the tutorial whenever they have free time) can be provided.

Training with the actual system is ideally done before implementation, since no real data have been collected. Users cannot accidentally change or erase actual data. Once the system has become operational, training becomes more difficult. It is difficult to train large numbers of people when access to data is limited to a small group of real patients. In addition, care must be taken to ensure the appropriate security of patient data. Consideration should be given to inventing hypothetical patients for training experiences.

Do not shortchange the training process. Allow for dedicated training time. Squeezing training in between a nurse's normal duties will only aid in frustrating new users. In addition, be sure to allow for training to occur over an extended period of time. Four two-hour sessions spread out over a one-week period are more beneficial than trying to perform eight hours of training in one day. Time is needed to digest the material.

Before a system becomes operational a period of system testing must occur. If the system is replacing a manual system, both the manual system and the computer system should be used simultaneously for at least a one- to three-month period. If the system is replacing an existing computerized system, then both computer systems should be used for a one- to three-month period.

Using both systems at once is known as *parallel operations.* Parallel operations cause a temporary decrease in productivity while both systems are being maintained. Therefore adequate planning is needed. The parallel operating period should never be used as the training period. Since individual workloads increase during parallel operations, frustration is often encountered. This frustration will be minimal if all users are adequately trained before parallel processing begins. Parallel operations should be limited to the shortest time period necessary to ensure the new system's reliability. Once the new system has proven itself the old system should be phased out.

Personnel. The successful development/implementation of an information system requires personnel who possess the following expertise: (1) the implementors must know what the system is needed to do, (2) the implementors must understand the generic issues that affect health care information systems, and (3) the implementors must be familiar with computer and communication technologies and have a feel for how these technologies will develop in the future. Because it is very rare to find individuals who possess expertise in all three areas, successful implementation of an information system must be a team effort.

The planning-phase team should consist of hospital users and systems personnel from the hospital's information system department. If adequate health care systems personnel are not available, outside systems consultants should be involved. At least one full-time nurse should be involved in any major nursing information system project (Steinberg and Toole, 1985). In addition, it is important to have several advisory committees representing key decision makers in the hospital. The nurse executive's role includes priority setting, allocating resources, choosing the right people for the project, providing space, and working toward plan acceptance (Carpenter, 1983).

In the project design phase nursing input is critical. A nursing advisory committee is responsible for providing feedback to the project team regarding evaluations of the management information system design, developing approaches for standardizing procedures at nursing stations, and developing long-term approaches to automating patient-care planning and other nursing functions (McCarthy, 1985). During the implementation phase, nurses, the hospital's information system department, and the hardware/software vendor must work closely together. Nurses who have a thorough understanding of current operating procedures must develop new guidelines for interfacing the new system with daily performed procedures. For example, in a patient-care system decisions as to which orders need verification must be made. This decision has a significant impact on system design and work flow.

Both systems personnel and nurses must work together to verify the accuracy of the system. Nurses are the only ones who can give systems personnel information on normal and peak-time activity. In addition nursing management must be intimately involved in scheduling formal training so as not to interrupt hospital operations.

Ingredients of Successful Implementation. Successful implementation depends on careful planning and analysis, commitment from administration at all levels, a team of individuals who work well together representing various departments and areas of expertise, and a little luck. More specifically:

1.   There must be strong administrative support at all levels of the hospital. Top-management commitment and enthu-

siasm for the new system affect user acceptance. If the system is seen as being extremely important for top management, and if enthusiasm for the new system is sensed, it is highly likely that the system will be successfully implemented. On the other hand, if top management is lukewarm or passively resists the new system, it is extremely unlikely that implementation will be successful. For systems that affect more than one service (that is, a patient-care system is accessed by nurses, physicians, pharmacists, and so on), it is extremely important that there be a rapport and cooperation among the departments.

2. If the system is to be developed in-house, experienced data processing staff dedicated to the project are essential.

3. The hospital must realize that significant resources will be required; these include financial resources (to purchase hardware/software and hire the necessary personnel), space, and time. Time and money for the education of participating staff must not be overlooked in system implementation.

4. There must be participation of key hospital personnel, including line and staff nurses. This is absolutely necessary for acceptance of the system. The participation should start at the beginning of the project in the needs analysis stage and continue through to system evaluation.

5. It is essential that there be realistic expectations as to what the system can do. A computer system cannot improve or replace bad management. In fact, if one is expecting that a computer system will improve bad management, it is highly likely that the system will make it worse. In addition, do not expect the system to be all things to all people. It is important to break down a large project into modules that are manageable.

6. Start with a system that will computerize an operation that is well understood and works well. Do not start with the worst problem you have. Implementing a computerized version of a well-organized and understood system is more likely to be successful. Once other members of the hospital staff see a system being successfully implemented, they will be more willing to computerize other operations that are more ambitious in scope.

7. Do not try to sell a computerized information system on the basis that you will need fewer personnel to perform the current tasks. More than likely you will need the same number of people, with only their responsibilities changing. Nurses will now be able to perform more patient care in a more efficient way. Instead of writing information into the chart, nurses or clerical workers will enter information into a computer. Clinical decisions will be made with better information, but "people power" is still required to do the thinking. As the responsibilities of nurses change, the information required will also change. It will be information technology's ability to manage the larger volume of clinical information that will allow the nurse to perform new functions.

8. Do not ask the information system to produce every conceivable report. You should ask yourself, "Why do I need the information?" Being selective in your information requests will enable the nurse manager to *use* the information.

9. Consideration should be given to terminal design and user interfaces. If a terminal is placed in an ergonomically appropriate position and the system is easy to learn and use, it will generally be well accepted.

Evaluation. Retrospective evaluation is often overlooked in the information system development/implementation process. Managing the development and implementation of an information system is very similar to implementing a planning process. Evaluating whether or not the plan, or in this case the information system, is meeting original goals and objectives is the only way an organization can learn whether or not the program was successful.

Work flows should be evaluated after the system becomes operational. Once a core group of patients have been entered, reports can be evaluated for their usefulness. In addition the overall efficiency of the system should be determined. These evaluations should occur after parallel operations have been completed.

The physical location and numbers of terminal and printers should be evaluated. It may seem as if additional terminals are needed to accommodate peak work periods, but alternatives in work flow might help to remedy any problems.

Software changes may be required if it is determined that work flow changes or different reports are required. These changes should be expected and are normal if users are utilizing the system. Work flow changes, if necessary, are harder to implement. Care should be taken not to develop too many artificial procedures that are difficult to follow, since staff will not accept these changes readily.

Success of the system can also be measured in terms of users' taking full advantage of its features. New users are often occupied with learning and utilizing the basic functions. If training is sufficient and the system well designed, it should not take long for users to take full advantage of each screen, function, and report.

Summary

Nurse executives are operating in an extremely competitive and rapidly changing high-technology environment. Computer technology is only one tool that can better enable nurse executives to manage these changes. Electronic software tools have the potential to make an executive's work easier and more efficient. Decision support systems with appropriate references to the hospital's management information systems provide a basis for sound decision making.

If it is determined that additional computerized systems are required to improve patient care or increase the efficiency of staff nurses, new or additional nursing information or hospital information systems can be implemented. A needs analysis must be completed and a request for proposal written. A vendor must be selected on the basis of the request for proposal, personal interviews, and reference checks. Implementation involves not only programming/installing the system but also formal training and parallel processing. As soon as implementation is initiated, a system evaluation process must be put into place to ensure that the information system is meeting the proposed system's objectives.

References

Blum, B. I., and Orthner, H. F. "Implementing Health Care Information Systems." In H. F. Orthner and B. I. Blum (eds.), *Implementing Health Care Information Systems.* New York: Springer-Verlag, 1986.

Carpenter, C. R. "Computer Use in Nursing Management." *Journal of Nursing Administration,* 1983, *13* (11), 17–21.

Drazen, E. L. "Planning for Purchase and Implementation of an Automated Hospital Information System: A Nursing Perspective." *Journal of Nursing Administration,* 1983, *13* (9), 9–12.

Entin, F. R. J. "Reviewing the Contract." *American Journal of Hospital Pharmacy,* 1982, *39* (8), 1324–1328.

Hicks, J. O. *Management Information Systems: A User Perspective.* New York: West, 1984.

McCarthy, L. "Taking Charge of Computerization." *Nursing Management,* 1985, *16* (7), 35–40.

Schmitz, H. H. *Managing Health Care Information Resources.* Rockville, Md.: Aspen, 1987.

Shelly, G. B., and Cashman, T. J. *Computer Fundamentals for an Information Age.* Brea, Calif.: Anaheim, 1984.

Steinberg, L., and Toole, J. "Role of a Systems Consultant During the Implementation of a Patient Care System." *Nursing Clinics of North America,* 1985, *20* (3), 567–575.

PART 3

People Skills
and Managing Behavior

CHAPTER 8

Managing People

Charles E. Dwyer

The Importance of Managing People

The basic, indeed the sole, reason for each of us to use any of our time and energy to interact with any organization, in any role whatsoever (for example, as employee, investor, supplier, client, regulator), is to see to it that the resources of that organization are used to take care of what is important to each of us. Since anything we might want from any organization is under someone's control, managing people is the primary function of all of our organizational activities.

Nearly everything that is important to us in our lives requires the cooperation of others. As a result, the quality of our lives is very much a function of our ability to influence people in myriad relationships.

One of the first and most common illusions people have about human influence is that some sort of magic is available to them—that there are some no-cost, no-risk, 100-percent-guaranteed ways of getting what we want from people. There are widespread convictions that we can acquire the newest fads from the leading business schools, from the most successful business organizations, or from the most prominent consulting organizations, insert them into our own organizations, and our problems will be magically solved. No such magic exists.

Those who want to be more effective with people must understand that substantial increases in effectiveness have substantial costs and risks. Those costs and risks are both subtle and ego-threatening, but if you are willing to accept them, there is virtually no limit to your potential for human influence. If you are not willing to accept them, then you must be content with your present level of influence, because it is unlikely to increase.

There is some good news in all of this. It is not difficult to understand, in most instances, what is necessary on your part to influence others. We have inappropriately and unnecessarily complicated and even mystified the requirements of human influence. Neither erudite knowledge nor special skill is needed. You already have most of the knowledge you need. Likewise, most of the skills you need are already available to you. Using the concepts presented in this chapter will enable you to gain more in a short period of time. Beyond that, all that is needed is a willingness to pay the price and assume the risks inherent in greatly increased effectiveness.

Values and Human Motivation

If you are to serve your values by tapping into the flow of organizational resources, if you are to have more power in organizations, if you are to influence behaviors more effectively, you must understand the role of values in human behavior—both your own values and those of others whom you wish to influence.

All behavior is designed (albeit subconsciously much of the time) to serve the values of the person who engages in it. People do not always select and execute their behaviors well, and therefore do not always manage to serve their values well; nonetheless, their intent is to take care of what is important to them. If you accept this concept, it can have profound implications for the ways you go about attempting to influence people. If people are attempting to serve their own values twenty-four hours a day, seven days a week, they will do what we want them to do only if they perceive that doing so will best serve their values. This quite simple point must be the basis for our efforts to influence others. If we look at both our successes and failures in influence, we discover that each can be well understood in terms of this basic tenet of human behavior.

At this point, a natural question arises: "How can I know what it is that people value?" There are several answers to this question, many of which will be dealt with later. For now, it is sufficient to recognize that there exists a basic set of values shared by nearly everyone, although with differing priorities, intensities, and concepts of how to serve them. These include a belief in the importance of or the need for self-esteem, acceptance, affiliation, friendship, security, freedom, autonomy, recognition, success, and fun. You have been influencing people since shortly after your birth, so you must have been touching others' values. As a result, you have a good sense of what is important to people (although perhaps not yet an explicit sense). At the same time, it is essential to recognize that all of us do not have identical value systems. We need to make discriminations, and in some cases we also need to read a given individual's value system with some precision. This, too, is possible.

The fact that all behavior is designed to serve the personal values of the person who engages in it does not imply that people are narrow, self-centered, or selfish in their behaviors. It simply means that each person is operating out of some sense of values in his or her own head. Those values may include altruism, morality, principles of ethics, and a sense of professionalism, duty, obligation, and concern for the welfare of others. The actions in support of these values are often painful and costly, but we do them with full knowledge of the risks to our narrower self-interest.

Power

Power is very much misunderstood, and many things that are thought to be sources of power are not. If you are to touch others' values in such a way as to influence their behavior, you must understand what power is in an organizational context.

Organizational Power. At its most elemental level, power is the ability to affect the allocation of organizational resources.

We each operate within (or interact with) an organization's resources. Since all organizational resources are under someone's control, organizational power is the ability to influence those people who have control.

Organizations have three functions and three elements. Their functions are to attract, transform, and then allocate resources in the form of value satisfactions to those who operate within and interact with the organization. The three elements of organizations are resources, people who are seeking value satisfactions from the organization, and power. Power is the organizational element that determines whose values will be served by organizational resources and how well they will be served.

Power and Authority. It is important to distinguish power from authority. Power is the ability to affect the allocation of resources. Authority is an organizationally granted privilege to engage in certain behaviors and expect to be supported in those activities—for example, to hire, fire, make policy, and direct procedures.

It is possible to have significant authority and little or no power. Likewise, it is possible to have no authority in a given organization but significant power. Certainly, substantial contributors to hospitals have no authority in the hospital, but they clearly have power when they and theirs come for treatment.

The Essence of Power. When all else is stripped away, we see that power, ultimately, is the ability to place certain quite specific perceptions in people's heads—perceptions that lead them to engage in the behaviors we want them to engage in. Others are doing what they do to take care of what is important to them—in order to serve their values. Our power depends on our ability to make them perceive that what *we* want them to do is the best thing they can do in the service of *their* values.

Communications researchers tell us that the average American adult is confronted with 350 to 700 messages per day trying to get through and influence behavior. Every ad, commercial billboard, bulletin board, newspaper article, piece of mail, phone call, and interpersonal encounter is filled with attempts to affect one's behavior. Since we cannot possibly deal on a conscious level with that flood of information, we create automatic screens to filter out most of it. At base, we use our values as the final screen; but since we cannot possibly give thoughtful consideration to every data point competing for our attention, we must erect superficial screens, at a subconscious level, to keep most things from ever reaching our conscious processing.

This has several implications for power. Basically, you must recognize that you are only one of the multitude of fragments of information or data points competing for the attention of those you are trying to influence. Often we overinvest in the power of our ideas, knowing how good they are and how effective for the organization, if only they are accepted and implemented. We know that truth, right, reason, evidence, and the facts are on our side. But none of this is relevant until someone pays attention. Even the truth and right are rarely, if ever, compelling.

An unhappy conclusion follows. We live in a world largely dependent on superficiality for effectiveness in human influence. Perceptions in people's heads are personal, subjective, fragile, and malleable states. They are often affected by shallow, nonsubstantive, and fleeting details and nuances. Those who try to sell us their goods and services are particularly aware of these relevant superficialities. The selection of a gesture, tone, or expression; the timing, placement, or pace of a television ad; the inclusion or exclusion of a word, a color, or texture—each is thought through consciously and is often agonized over. Advertisers know that they have little time and only a slim chance of getting through to us.

Anyone who wishes to increase his or her effectiveness in managing people must think in a similar way. Such an approach feels awkward. We are not accustomed to thinking through our words and gestures, our timing, and our approach. To do so seems unnatural and forced. We are accustomed to doing what feels most comfortable—usually only things that seem reasonable and persuasive to us.

Rationalization

If you are to change your behavior and become more effective, you will need to rid yourself of certain patterns—patterns placed

there early in life by the culture and patterns that you have
repeated thousands of times. In essence, those patterns control
your present behavior and act as monumental bars to managing people.

A Cultural "Gift." When we were three- or four-year-olds,
we were faced with a difficult problem. We tried to influence
someone and failed to do so. We suffered feelings of frustration, anger, disappointment, and even rage. Such failures had
occurred many times before, but at age three our negative feelings were intensified because the culture began to teach us that
failure is a negative outcome, an assault on our self-esteem. At
about the same time, we learned that we were supposed to have
reasons for our emotions and for our successes and failures. We
began to need these reasons, not just for our parents but also
within our heads. We learned to manufacture them.

Between the ages of three and four we also learned the
importance of feeling good about ourselves. We wanted to be
accepted rather than rejected. We wanted to be approved of.
And then the problem arose for us. We each tried to get someone to let us have something we wanted (for example, a toy,
to stay up later, to go to the zoo), and we failed to influence
that person. The familiar rush of negative emotions rolled over
us, intensified by the newly discovered need to avoid failure.
But now we also needed a reason for our negative emotions.
We did not want to think that the reason we had failed was that
we were undeserving. We needed a reason that was acceptable
to us in terms of approval and positive self-esteem.

Now, finding such a reason is a rather sophisticated task
for a three-year-old child. But a culture that makes a demand
tends to give an answer, and this case is no exception. We each
learned to respond to such situations by saying both aloud and
to ourselves (preferably with clenched fists and teeth), "NOT
FAIR, NOT FAIR!" This response met our criteria. It provided
a reason that was often accepted by others, and it put blame
outside ourselves. At three, we had very little understanding
of justice and fairness. Nonetheless, we knew how to project
blame and scapegoat the world for what we did not like in our

lives. We begin saying "not fair" at about age three and a half, and most of us continue the refrain for the rest of our lives.

As we mature into our teenage years, we develop variations on the theme. Now we blame our negative emotions and failures on the defects of our parents, who "don't understand us," "don't care about us," and "don't trust us." This is precisely the same behavior as the three-year-old's.

This set of behaviors runs its course by the time we are in our early to mid twenties. We continue to experience the same failures and emotions, but our parents are no longer constraining our behavior. That makes them implausible scapegoats. But we still need reasons so we shift to other targets. "It's the system, the bureaucracy, the red tape, the establishment!" "It's those intractable, intransigent, insensitive, irresponsible, stupid, negative, impossible people I have to work with!"

In all these cases we are rationalizing—lying to ourselves. In doing so, we are reducing our effectiveness. Each of us has limited time and energy to serve our values. Time spent in rationalizing is time *not* spent in influencing others.

Our lack of substantial effectiveness in influencing people is less a function of our failed attempt than it is a function of our failure to try to influence or to persist. To try to influence or to persist in the face of rejection is to risk failure. To rationalize is to enjoy the comfort, ease, security, and support of a well-known place.

An Alternative Program. Much has been learned in recent years about how programming takes place in our brains. There are two principal mechanisms: experience of a significant emotional event and repetition. Repetition is by far the more common.

We have also learned that we can eliminate the influence of a program on us by substituting a new program for it—a more powerful program that overrides the old one. An example: NEVER EXPECT ANYONE TO ENGAGE IN A BEHAVIOR THAT SERVES YOUR VALUES UNLESS YOU GIVE THAT PERSON ADEQUATE REASON TO DO SO!

When this new program plays in your head, it will impel

you to seek solutions. It will drive you to action rather than to rationalization. The new program states a proposition I believe you will agree with. First, if someone is doing something you do not want them to do or is failing to do something you want them to do, do you think their behavior makes sense to them? Of course it does. Our behaviors always make sense to us. And people do not change their behaviors unless they have some reason to do so.

What constitutes "adequate reason"? Adequate reason is what works. Adequate reason does not mean that you argue with people or present them with facts and other data, though it may include evidence and logic. More broadly, it means using your behavior to help people make connections in their heads that are not presently there. Behavior is a function of perceptions, and perceptions are what you must shape.

Installing a New Program

If you know how to drive a car, you know what an automatic program is. No doubt you have been out on a highway and suddenly realized that you have traveled twenty-five miles without paying any conscious attention to your driving. While panic may have momentarily seized you, you did, nonetheless, survive those twenty-five miles. You were operating on automatic. A subconscious program was controlling your behavior. If the brake lights of a vehicle in front of you had lit up, your brain would have picked up the data from your eyes and sent a signal to your leg and foot to step on the brake.

That automatic driving program was not always there. When we first learn to drive, it seems difficult, and we wonder if we will ever learn properly. While learning, we have to pay conscious attention to every detail, and it seems that there are more details than we are able to manage. But we keep on, repetition finally does its job, and we produce the program.

To break an automatic program we must first bring it up to consciousness. There is a specific method you must follow if you are to succeed in doing this. If you have ever driven in a country with a reversed steering wheel location, such as

England or Ireland, you know what it is like to have the wrong program. You found that the "natural" way of doing things is illegal, counterproductive, even suicidal. But if you persisted for a few days and consciously practiced the new way of driving, you found that you were able to install a new program that overrode the old one. The old one was still there, however, and on returning home you were able to connect with it quickly.

The same can be done with our tendency to rationalize in situations of human influence. The override program can be installed so that it plays in place of the old scapegoating program.

In England or Ireland, there are distinct advantages available to us in installing the new driving program. For one, we have extremely high motivation to do so, given the consequences of our failure to do so. Next, we are constantly bombarded with visual cues, reminding us of the dysfunctionality of our old program and the requirements of the new one. The steering wheel is in an unfamiliar place; road signs are on the left; we see other cars approach on our right. We are bombarded with signs telling us what the new program is, and we become very sensitive to them.

In terms of our nonrationalization program, we are at a distinct disadvantage. Not only do we not have any cues in our environment reminding us to install the new program, but all the relevant cues are in the opposite direction. We are surrounded by people who want us to rationalize, who will invite us to do so, and who will support us in our efforts — all because they will later call on us to help them rationalize.

This means that we have to create our own cues — cues to remind us of the new program and to practice it. Otherwise we do not bring the old one up to consciousness; and if we do not, it will not change.

Often people believe that because they understand the desirability of a change in their lives, it will take place. That is simply not how our brains function. Have you ever been angry in some interpersonal relationship and found, after you cooled down, that your anger was both foolish and counterproductive? Probably you resolved not to get angry again in that kind of situation. But chances are that as soon as you found yourself in that situation again (that is, the cues appeared), you became angry, despite your best intentions to the contrary and despite the action of your willpower. We cannot *will away* any of our programs.

In installing the new nonrationalization program, some of the following suggestions may be helpful to you. They will make it easier to bring it up to consciousness for repetition. Print the new program out in large letters on an 8½-by-11-inch sheet of paper, make several copies, and then put them in places where they are certain to attract your attention, for example, in an often used closet or drawer, framed on the wall of your office, or taped to some prominent place in your car. (You may have to move them occasionally, or the brain, as an energy conservation mechanism, will cease to notice them consciously. Unless they are placed where you must "trip over" them on the way to something else, you will "learn" to overlook them, just as you usually overlook the furniture in your home.) You should simultaneously imagine the situations that currently trigger rationalization and see and hear yourself saying the new program.

Memorization of the statement is not the goal. That can be done in a few seconds. The objective is to have several cues per day to remind you, at a conscious level, to rehearse the statement imaginatively so that it will override the old program. Within about two weeks the new statement should start to interfere with the old program of rationalization in the rehearsed situation. After that, it should begin to dominate. Do not be discouraged if, on occasion, the old programs play. This just proves that they are still there.

Once a new program is installed, the primary issue switches to methods: what to do to supply adequate reason to influence the behavior of others. This requires focusing on the issue of perceptions—those personal, subjective, fragile, and malleable states in people's heads that control their behaviors.

Mistakes in Human Influence. People who recognize the connection between values and behavior often make a serious mistake. They assume a one-to-one correlation, that is, if people have certain values, they will thereby engage in certain behaviors. Because it neglects the critical role of *perceptions,* this assumption leads to errors in managing people.

The most serious of these errors results when we assess and serve the values of those we wish to influence with the expectation that they will then engage in the desired behavior. We often heap value satisfactions on people (for example, salary, bonuses, fringe benefits, and improved working conditions), hoping that they will feel gratitude and give us a desired behavior in return. Such a system simply does not work.

We tend to blame these individuals for not doing what we want. Why should they? It is apparent to them that we are willing to give, without getting in return.

Perceptions, Values, and Behaviors. What you want someone to do is *irrelevant* in his or her decision. What is critical is that person's *perception of the relationship between what you want that person to do and that person's values.* This is the necessary connection within that person's head. This is the personal, subjective, fragile, and malleable state that controls behavior. See Figure 8.1.

Figure 8.1. The Connection Between Values and Behavior.

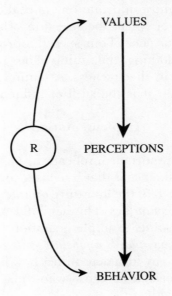

Perhaps, at a given time in your life, you were absolutely sure that there was a certain behavior you would never, ever engage in, yet later you did. The connection in your head between that behavior and your values changed.

Human influence entails getting someone else to see something that makes sense to that person. What makes sense to him or her may not make sense to you and vice versa. Each person is unique, with his or her own personal values, beliefs, experiences, ways of processing information, and so on. If you fail the first time to get what you want, there is no reason to become either defensive or discouraged. People are complex. Another approach is called for. If it does not succeed, yet another may work; and yet another again may be required before the connection is made.

Images. The dominance of perceptions in human influence implies another need: Each of us must become more sensitive to the details of our own behavior. Since we are dealing with personal and subjective states in others' heads, very small differences in what we do can make very large differences in perceptions and in our effectiveness. As noted, people have filters and screens that keep most information out of their processing programs. Our tone of voice, the selection of a single word, the rhythm, volume, or pace of our speech, our gestures and facial expressions, our clothing, the timing of our request — each may play a critical role in effectiveness. Attention to such detail may be bothersome, but it is the stuff of influence.

Implementation

One of the most important implications of the role of perceptions in human influence is that it focuses concentration on implementation. Much of the literature on management attempts to evaluate which techniques of human influence work and which do not. Analysis points to implementation: *One hundred percent of the effectiveness of any idea is a function of its implementation.* The implementation of any idea determines how it will be perceived; and how it is perceived by those who must cooperate with it determines its effectiveness.

But most people are tempted to attribute the success or failure of an idea to the idea itself. They search in vain for "successful" ideas. Surely, some ideas are more easily implemented than others, but the key issue is still implementation.

There is a tendency to reject the importance of implementation because it places responsibility for failure squarely on the person doing the implementing. We would much prefer to conclude that an ineffective implementation is the result of a bad idea rather than a flawed implementation. The centrality of implementation also reminds us of the futility of the search for magic in managing people. The prepackaged "solution" to our people problems does not and cannot exist, because the implementation of the idea fully determines its success or failure.

The Costs of Effectiveness

Several of the costs and risks of being effective in managing people have already been noted: assuming responsibility for one's own effectiveness; giving up the comfort of warm, secure, easy, habitual, well-worn, and well-supported rationalizations; confronting one's own failures and fears of failure; and facing accusations resulting from treating people differently. But there are other significant costs and risks.

Behaviors That Feel Good Are Often Not Effective. Many of the behaviors we engage in on a daily basis deliver an immediate satisfaction to us. We eat a meal, watch a ball game, or go to a movie because such behaviors are immediately enjoyable. See Figure 8.2.

Many of our behaviors also involve other people, but influence is not always our primary reason for engaging in them. Our primary motivation is often the immediate satisfaction they give us. The behavior itself serves our values, independent of the impact on the other person. For example, we may do a favor for a friend more to bolster our self-image as a friend than to influence the friend's future behavior. Our behavior may influence that friend's future behavior — indeed, any behavior in which we engage in the presence of others (or that reaches them in any way) has some effect on them; but many of these behaviors

Figure 8.2. The Choices Between Behaviors
That Feel Good and Behaviors That Are Effective.

TRADE-OFFS

CHOICES

CONFLICTS

PRIORITIES

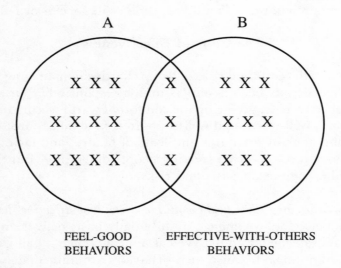

FEEL-GOOD   EFFECTIVE-WITH-OTHERS
BEHAVIORS   BEHAVIORS

have as their primary motivation the satisfaction immediately
derived.

Most of these behaviors are easy for us to engage in because they feel good, and our satisfaction (or value serving) is
delivered by the behaviors that are also effective in influencing
the behavior of others. Therefore, we must move to the effective set of behaviors, and those, for the most part, do not feel
good; they have costs and risks for us.

Effective Behaviors Often Do Not Feel Good. Thus one of
the primary reasons each of us is not more effective in influenc-

ing others is because we are unwilling to do what is necessary. Even though the behaviors are easily available and we have known about them most of our lives, we do not use them because they have personal costs and risks.

For example, one of the most powerful influential behaviors ever invented is a *request for help*. If you are asked for help and the person requesting it does not "overdo it," you feel flattered. You have been given power in the relationship. You can reject the request. You have been offered partial ownership of the task (how much easier it is to suggest how things should be done when you are a participant rather than a spectator). You are being offered some probable recognition and gratitude. You are being identified as someone who is altruistic, as someone who will give help to others. And if you give the requested help, the other person "owes" you. You can feel good about yourself and "put money in the bank" at the same time — it is much easier to ask someone for help if you have recently given that person help. You are not becoming indebted. You are simply "righting" the scales of justice.

These are just some of the reasons why asking for help is a powerful approach to human influence. Why don't we do more of it? Because the same elements of asking for help that make it powerful make us reluctant to use it. We do not want to make ourselves vulnerable to rejection; we do not want to reinforce our dependencies on others; we do not want to share ownership; we do not want to share credit; we do not want to become indebted. And so, when we want something from another, we do not ask for help. Rather we are likely to say something like, "*We* have a problem!" — a safe approach, but one that has very little chance of being effective. If we get what we want, we owe nothing. There is no vulnerability; there is no asymmetry in the relationship. If we do not get what we want, we can always fault the other for "not knowing how serious this problem really is." We refuse to do what works because we are unwilling to pay the freight.

Perhaps, on occasion, you have said something like the following: "I have done everything possible to deal with her and nothing works." Operationally this sentence usually means: "I tried a couple of safe, comfortable things that felt good, and they didn't work, so it must be her!" As a check, analyze situations where you feel you have tried everything. Recall whether or not you asked that person for help. Chances are that you did not do so. Therefore you did not do "everything possible."

Giving recognition is frequently as powerful as asking for help. People are starved for recognition. Recognition is powerful precisely because it gives people something they value in exchange for behavior helpful to you. It significantly increases the likelihood that they will repeat that behavior in the future. Unfortunately, the far more common refrain heard from people in most organizations is "When I do it right, I hear nothing. When I do it wrong, I hear *everything*."

Recognition is in short supply. Why? It seems that for most people, giving recognition is not a feel-good behavior. It is perceived as having costs and risks for the user: "If I give her recognition, she will ask for more money or look for a better job." "He will think he is better than he is." "She will get the credit for the effectiveness of my department." "If you give too much recognition you cheapen the currency." "I don't get recognition for what I do. Why should my people get it from me?"

There are real costs and risks in giving recognition, but we generally seem to overstate them in order to rationalize not doing something we really do not feel comfortable doing. If you want to achieve an instant increase in effectiveness, get in the habit of *writing* two or three brief notes of appreciation and recognition *per week* to those in and around your organization. Watch the changes in their behavior toward you. I guarantee they will become even more anxious to please you in the hope of getting such recognition again.

Each of us knows the easiest, most powerful way to have an idea accepted and implemented by a superior: let the superior take ownership and credit for the idea. Then why not use it? "Because," we say, "it's not fair. It's my idea. I should get credit for it." Fair or not, feel good or not, letting superiors take credit is very effective.

Some "Feel-Good" Behaviors Interfere with Effectiveness.
If you want substantially increased effectiveness, you not only must take on a number of risky and costly behaviors, but you

must also give up some behaviors you find very satisfying. Each of us has values we serve on a daily basis—values we would prefer not to admit to ourselves, such as dominance, deference, superiority, self-indulgence, and aggression. These values give rise to multiple behaviors: interruptions of subordinates, unnecessary commands, dominations of meetings we chair, ventings of frustrations, and so on. Such behaviors have impacts on those at whom they are directed and on others who become aware of them. They affect their perceptions, attitudes, and subsequent behaviors. Those subsequent behaviors are unlikely to be supportive of our values.

This is not to suggest that we are all egomaniacs and wait anxiously for opportunities to pounce on the unsuspecting. Rather, it suggests that each of us is susceptible to being captured by the attraction of the natural value satisfiers for managers in hierarchical organizations.

Fear of Failure. Still another impediment to effectiveness in human influence is fear of failure. It has been put into each of us, by our culture, at an early age. In attempting to influence anyone (outside of the easy, almost guaranteed conventions we use on a daily basis), we run the risks of failure, rejection, and embarrassment. We have been taught to avoid these risks. They constitute assaults on the most precious and well protected of our values—self-esteem. We do not want to "look bad" either in our own eyes or in the eyes of others. Our lack of effectiveness in managing people is less a consequence of our failures than it is a consequence of our reluctance to try in the first place.

Most of the effective techniques for human influence require that you make the first move and accept vulnerabilty to failure. Effectiveness requires persistence through rejections and repeated failures. To acquire such persistence we must overcome well-worn beliefs about failure and well-worn emotional programs that have played thousands of times in our heads.

The Values Approach

Earlier we explored the idea that you should never expect anyone to engage in a behavior that serves your values unless you give that person "adequate reason" to do so. "Adequate reason" means linking, *in that person's perception,* the behavior (or behavioral outcome) you want to that person's values. There are two general ways of accomplishing that linking: the positive approach and the negative approach. This section will focus on one of those ways, the positive approach.

The Positive Approach. The positive approach to human influence consists of a five-part model of human information processing. It constitutes a set of lenses each of us can use to increase our repertoire of behaviors in managing people. It is a template that can be used in any attempt to influence another person. If the interrelated conditions are met, you can get anyone to do anything you want.

1. *Capability.* The first item a potential influencee is likely to process in any attempt to influence his or her behavior is his or her capability. Capability consists of three elements:

- Does the person know what *behavior* or behavioral outcome is sought? Sometimes people do not do what we want them to do because they simply do not know in adequate detail what it is that is being asked of them.
- Does the person have the *competence* to engage in the desired behavior? Competence includes knowledge, skill, talent, other personal resources, and the opportunity necessary to engage in the behavior.
- Does the person have the necessary *confidence* in his or her competence to engage in the behavior? Confidence is one's perception of one's own competence. Sometimes people who are competent by all objective measures are difficult to influence because they do not have the requisite confidence. Because of our fears of failure, confidence is a necessary component in any undertaking. (It is also possible for someone to be highly confident and yet incompetent. Such a person will try anything, fail, and then rationalize the failure.)

There are two kinds of errors we make with respect to the issue of capability. We can underestimate people's capabilities, thereby missing opportunities because we fail to try to influence them. If they are aware of our underestimation of their capabilities, we may also offend them and stimulate accompanying negative behavior.

The second error is to overestimate capabilities. In this case we try to influence someone and fail. We invest our time and energy in an unproductive way. Furthermore, when someone who lacks capability is the subject of influence, he or she often reacts negatively to the influencer. It is awkward to be asked to do something you cannot (or believe you cannot) do. The intended influencee is unlikely to try the behavior and risk failure, nor will this person admit incompetence. The result is someone who gives excuses, procrastinates, and otherwise engages in unproductive behaviors in order to hide his or her lack of capability. The least productive action the influencer can take in such a situation is to press the person, since this will lead to increasingly defensive and potentially bizarre behavior, thereby stimulating more pressure from the influencer and still more defensive behavior, in an ever-worsening cycle of negative interpersonal relationships.

This condition is the "can" condition, and if not met, there is no point in going further, because no amount of willingness can make up for a lack of capability. If you suspect that the person you are trying to influence is lacking in capability, you have several options open to you:

- Look for an alternative behavior that the person is capable of.
- Team the person up with another to create combined capability.
- Look for someone else to do it.
- Do it yourself.
- Increase the person's capability.
- Forget it and find some other way to serve your values.

Not all of these options are feasible in all situations, but many are overlooked when they are viable owing to our egos. Our egos insist that we "make" *that* person engage in *that* behavior.

At this given point a person is capable of a wide range

of behaviors: He or she *can* do many things. What he or she *will* do is a function of the ways in which the next four conditions are processed in that person's perceptions.

2. *Perception of Potential Value Satisfaction.* People do what they do to take care of their values. Anyone you are to influence (at least in terms of the positive approach) must perceive something of value to them in the behavior. If the perception is not already there, then you must put it there.

The following list includes many of the common values of Americans:

Principles

Justice	"Morality"	Sense of obligation/duty
Honesty	"Righteousness"	Truth
Equality	Beauty	

Values Used to Serve Others

Caring for	Sharing with	Responsibility for
Concern about	Interest in	Protecting
Security of	Loving	Bringing happiness to
Being of help to	Friendship	Acceptance of
Kindness	Compassion	Open-mindedness
Being of service to	Patience	Consideration
Understanding		

Values Served by Others

Affiliation	Being needed	Dependence
Friendship	Sense of community	Interdependence
Love	Working together	Admiration
Acceptance	Appreciation	Compliments
Understanding	Recognition	Approval
Togetherness	Status	Gratitude
Sharing	Esteem	Loyalty
Giving	Praise	Opposition
Companionship	Deference	Tolerance
Consideration	Cooperation	Attention
Thoughtfulness	Commitment	

Inner Values

Security	Wisdom/knowledge	Competition
Health	Learning	Fun
Self-satisfaction	Harmony	Humor
Self-esteem	Success/achievement	Contentment
Self-control	Advancement	Happiness
Self-respect	Power	Peace of mind

Self-value	Curiosity	Sense of well-being
Pride/dignity	Autonomy	Skill
Significance	Freedom	Comfort
Independence	Sense of commitment	Relaxation
Challenge	Excitement	Recreation
	Being right	Pleasure

This list contains few surprises. Both by introspection and by the lifelong observation of people's behavior, we know a great deal about people's values. Effectiveness is primarily a matter of codifying and formalizing our knowledge. If you reflect for a moment, you will realize that you already know a great deal about how to serve (or threaten) the values of nearly any one of the 5 billion people on the face of the earth. You know that people want to feel good about themselves, to feel secure, to receive recognition, esteem, respect, and status, to have security, autonomy, and fun, to achieve, to be deferred to, to have power, to be admired, and so on. Again, it is a matter of our unwillingness to give them these satisfactions *in return for the behavior we want from them* that keeps us from effectively using our considerable knowledge.

We know that it is possible to read people's values. As we observe people or as we analyze their behavior retrospectively, we can often begin to see patterns of values emerge. Asking others who know the person better than we do can also offer insights. Sometimes the people themselves can be approached and are willing to reveal some of what is important to them. Try looking at one of the columns of values in the preceding list. Put a particular person in mind; then, using a scale of minus 5 to plus 5, indicate the various weights that you believe are representative of the force of those values in that person's life. You have drawn a value profile of that person. You may be surprised at how much you already know.

3. *Perception of Probability of Value Satisfaction.* Once people see some potential value satisfaction in a situation of influence, the next issue is their perception of the *probability* of receiving that satisfaction. For the most part, this has to do with levels of *trust*. To what extent does the potential influencee believe that the value satisfaction will be received after the sought-after be-

havior has been carried out? No matter how high the perceived value, it is worthless if the perceived probability of getting it is nil. Trust is enormously powerful and equally fragile. People will do things for people they trust that they would do for no one else. But trust is like Humpty Dumpty—once broken it is very difficult to put back together.

We need to be consistent and follow through. We need to deliver on what we promise, and we must subtly let people know that we will deliver. There are few, if any, actions more powerful than building a reputation of trust.

The perceived probability of value satisfaction is so important that it has occupied the minds of influencers (particularly in situations of desired influence but little or no trust) as long as there have been people. In past times, it gave rise to the practice of exchanging hostages. More recently, it is responsible for the development of contract law, security deposits, and escrow accounts—each a substitute for interpersonal trust. These arrangements allow people who do not know and/or trust one another to influence one another. Each arrangement embodies a common principle of human influence. We put something of great value at risk (even under the control of the influencee), and it is forfeited if we fail to deliver the promised value satisfaction. This process does not feel good, but it is very effective in managing people.

4. *Perception of Cost.* Whenever you wish to influence anyone, that person will perceive a cost in doing what you want of him or her. It may be nothing more than the time and energy involved in doing it. It may be that the person (rightly or wrongly) perceives that doing what you want will cost in terms of friendships, family relationships, or job opportunities. Whether such perceptions are accurate or in any way realistic is beside the point. Such perceptions keep people from doing what we want. Therefore, altering perceived cost is another technique for achieving greater influence.

5. *Perception of Risk.* Some value satisfactions are thought certain to be lost if a behavior is engaged in. These represent perceptions of cost. Those we wish to influence are also concerned about other value satisfactions that *might* be threatened

or lost. These constitute the influencee's *perception of risk*. There may be several potential risks, and the influencee will assign varying subjective probabilities to each of them. Generally, the most important are loss of self-esteem, rejection, failure, embarrassment, "looking bad," disapproval, greater cost than originally thought, and vague uncertainty that something might "go wrong." Perceived risks are a powerful element of potential influence, but their vagueness and subjectivity make them difficult to influence.

The influencer tends almost inevitably to inflate the potential value satisfaction and probability of value satisfaction of the influencee and to discount his or her *perceived* cost and risk. At the same time, the influencee has a strongly reinforced cultural tendency to react in the opposite way — to discount perceived potential value satisfaction and probability of value satisfaction and to inflate perceived cost and risk. The influencer wants to be persuasive *and* to appear reasonable in his or her own mind; the influencee has been burned before and is cautious. The person who wishes to influence others must be aware of these opposing tendencies and be prepared to compensate for them.

The influencer must affect the weightings given the five conditions by the influencee. Each increase in perceived potential value satisfaction and probability of value satisfaction moves the influencee toward the behavior, as does each decrease in perception of cost or risk. The goal is to affect the weightings sufficiently so that the influencee will move across the threshold to the positive side and decide to engage in the behavior.

A potential influencee can be visualized as being on the left or negative side of a continuum. It may require several moves before the influencee perceives "adequate reason," that is, before he or she moves over to the positive side.

Thousands of moves that have an impact on perception are visible all around us. We need only put on the proper lenses to find them and evaluate them, then select those that are most likely to be useful to us in our organizations.

How to Use the Model. There are several ways in which the model can be used to build a much more powerful personal repertoire of effective behaviors for influencing others.

1. Use it when you fail, not to look for what you did wrong but to discover what you might have done differently to improve the probability of success. Learn from failure. Focusing on learning also helps to reduce the likelihood that you will engage in either self-pity or rationalization.

2. Use it when you meet resistance. Using the model can leverage your next attempt. Persistence in the face of resistance is highly desirable; but intelligent persistence, based on concepts of how to alter the influencee's perceptions, is far superior.

3. Use it when you have a highly important instance of influence, and you have some planning time. Exactly what are you going to do? How? When? Where? Use it to plan presentations. Design your presentations around the perceptions and values of your audience. Precisely how have you designed your behavior to put the appropriately weighted perceptions in the minds of those you wish to influence?

4. Use it when you succeed in influencing someone, particularly when that person offered initial resistance. Learn from your successes. What did you do that brought the person across the threshold? Can it be repeated?

5. Use it when someone succeeds in influencing you, particularly when you offered initial resistance. What did that person do to influence you? What brought you across the threshold? Can you learn from it and use it in other settings?

6. Use it whenever you observe an instance of impressive influence. We all witness many instances of unusually effective influence. Some people in every organization are markedly better than others at getting what they want. You now have a tool for evaluating their successes. Furthermore, we are confronted with ads and promotions that we recognize as being extremely successful even though we do not use the product or service. We can examine these successful instances of influence and learn from them.

To be sure, even when we use the model we will always be guessing, that is, making judgments. But they will be informed guesses, aided by an understanding of the way in which people process information and decide (albeit usually subconsciously) to do or not to do whatever you are trying to get them to do.

Conclusions

A little knowledge, a little skill, and a great deal of willingness to pay costs and to take risks can yield substantial improvements in one's effectiveness in managing people. Few dimensions of the quality of our lives are as critical as our success in influencing the behavior of others. People do what they do in order to take care of what is important to them, that is, to serve their values. Power is the ability to influence the allocation of an organization's resources. It is the ability to place certain quite specific perceptions — personal, subjective, fragile, and malleable states — in other people's heads.

You have been enculturated to defend your ego from failure and to explain your negative emotions in terms of things external to you — to lie to yourself. Never expect anyone to engage in a behavior that serves your values unless you give that person adequate reason to do so. Behavior is a function of values mediated by perceptions. It is possible to get anyone to do anything you want, but in some cases the actions required may cost more than you are willing to pay.

The power you have to influence others is totally dependent on your behavior. You must give up rationalizing, subject yourself to charges of unfairness, take on costly and risky behaviors, and overcome your deeply entrenched fear of failure in order to increase your effectiveness in managing people.

People you are trying to influence process the data of your attempts to influence them in terms of their capability, perception of potential value satisfaction, perception of probability of value satisfaction, perception of cost, and perception of risk. This model constitutes a set of lenses. These lenses can be used in multiple contexts to greatly increase your repertoire of effective behaviors in influencing others.

References

Cialdini, R. *Influence: How and Why People Agree to Things.* New York: Morrow, 1984.

Cohen, A. R., and Bradford, D. *Influence Without Authority.* New York: Wiley, 1990.

Fisher, R., and Ury, W. *Getting to Yes: Negotiating Agreement Without Giving In.* Boston: Houghton Mifflin, 1981.

CHAPTER 9

Building and Maintaining Effective Working Alliances

Thomas North Gilmore

In hospitals and health care organizations, competitive pressures are dramatically increasing interdependence among functions, levels, and roles. The era of "loose coupling" is over (Weick, 1976). The costs of having a few days go by before social services finds an acceptable nursing home for a patient ready to leave are too great. Linking innovative dietary approaches to radiation therapy is critical to creating a competitive edge for oncology "products." Capital dollars are too limited to overbuild the number of operating rooms as a way of preventing conflicts among surgeons in scheduling the OR.

As health care grows increasingly specialized, those institutions that can effectively manage interdependence will have a distinct competitive advantage. As a customer orientation comes to be taken seriously, health care organizations will have to attend to the integration of various services to create a satisfactory experience for both patient and family. Quality service is dependent on the linkages among specific episodes, especially since each employee both sets expectations for the next step and shapes the perception of previous episodes. If these transitions are poorly managed, a patient may be dissatisfied even though each component was technically good work. Like music, the meaning for a customer may come as much from the spaces in between the notes as from the notes themselves.

As with other organizations in the ever-growing service sector, hospitals have rushed to embrace popular texts that preach excellence and customer orientation (Peters and Waterman, 1982; Peters and Austin, 1985). But what is written in a mission statement or advertising campaign cannot be realized without the work relationships necessary to implement the strategy. The link with the nurse executive is the channel into the largest and most pervasive group in the hospital. He or she carries the culture and is on the critical boundary with patients. In a fundamental way almost everyone in a hospital works on nursing's territory. With increased outpatient testing and surgery, the primary reason for admission to a hospital will be the need for nursing care. The CEO's confidence in the nurse executive and the quality of their working alliance will be critical in setting the tone for the institution. The nurse executive must balance the dilemmas of being at the same time the leader of a professional and clinical department and a full member of the executive team. The former role propels one to identify vertically with the nursing group; the latter, horizontally with all the others who interact with nursing. Part of the difficulty in managing the array of working alliances is the psychological strain of multiple identifications. It may be easier to feel fully aligned with nursing, even joining in the often belabored struggles with physicians, than to experience the confusing loyalties of multiple work relationships.

In this chapter I will begin by looking at the role constellations of nursing and the way new strategic challenges are both straining and strengthening these relationships. In the second section, I will look at some of the underlying anxieties that often distort the capacity for work across levels and roles. In the third section, I will examine the exchange of role perceptions in three dimensions: up, down, and laterally. Here I will introduce the structured process of role negotiation as a vehicle for clarifying working relationships. Then, in the fourth section, I will address ways to increase the quality of group thinking. In the fifth section, I will introduce a second structured technique — responsibility charting — for negotiating roles and responsibilities. In the last section, I will give advice on the repairing, building, and maintaining of effective work relationships in the complex, fast-changing setting of hospitals.

The Role Constellation of the Nurse Executive

A chief nursing officer must maintain working alliances with a network of key others. The span of control issues within the department pales in comparison to the active network with key others that must be maintained (see Figure 9.1). Nor are these relationships static. They are being dramatically strained, strengthened, or weakened by the following strategic challenges in health care.

Figure 9.1. Role Relationships of Nurse Executive.

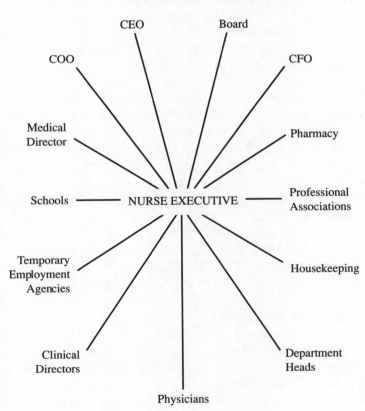

Diminished Resources. Shifts in reimbursements and fiscal constraints are increasing the interdependence of nursing and administration, raising difficult issues of nursing productivity. Nursing costs may be one of the hardest hit during retrenchment. Some see a regression for nursing with more pressure to reassume functions that nursing had delegated to others, such as respiratory therapy and IV teams. One CEO commented that "we have not yet defined the nursing product, and in the absence of that definition, we all too often fall into seeing their role through the doctors' eyes. We need to define clinical outcomes for nursing. We have given them accountability for a budget, but not for a product." Another noted that when he suggested the use of nurse aides for certain tasks such as bed baths, nursing might justify their need to hold on to that task because they are "assessing the psychosocial needs of the patient while giving the bath." These issues make it difficult to reach decisions that have quality-cost trade-offs.

Organizational Changes. New corporate forms of organization, redefinitions of divisions, into product lines, for example, and the increased focus on alternatives outside the hospital (for example, day surgery and home health care) change relationships among the top team. Corporate structures often remove the nurse executive from adequate contact with the CEO, who must now oversee a larger, more complex system. Alternatively, if the top nursing official gets pulled into the wider array of issues, he or she risks losing the necessary contact with the nursing organization. The result may be the loss of clinical leadership of the largest and most important department in the hospital. Combined with the preceding trend toward diminished resources, many hospitals have thinned the management ranks and given oversight of ancillary services to nursing. For example, social services, pharmacy, and respiratory therapy increasingly may be under nursing. This raises dilemmas for both the nurse executive and the chief executive in that it can have a paradoxical effect: By increasing the scope of nursing, the function may get diluted with concerns in other areas.

Marketing and Customer Trends. The marketing and customer trends make the nursing organization critical because nursing shapes so much of the customer's experience. This makes nursing more important. As one CEO, in discussing who the top nursing officer should report to, said, "It's the critical department, the two-thirds of the budget, responsible for half of the house, at the critical bedside. It's more than enough to be 'only responsible' for nursing and to be reporting directly to the CEO and be the most important member of the top team."

Anxieties in Work Relationships

In this section, I want to touch on certain underlying anxieties that often distort effective working relationships. Each of us as adults carries into our work relationships primitive thoughts and feelings that can disturb and distort the accomplishing of work (Segal, 1985). The following types of anxiety seem to be particularly at play in work relationships in a hierarchy.

Anxieties About Aggression. Anxieties about aggression are especially rampant in the context of supervision. The fear is that we will be too harsh, too mean, too tough, that in fantasy we might destroy the other persons, or so provoke them that they would retaliate. Aggression is necessary to do work. However, the fear that there is an excess, beyond what the task requires, provokes considerable anxiety. This is furthered because we inevitably have stored up resentments and irritations, and when there is an occasion for discharging these feelings, we sometimes fear that we will lose control and overwhelm the other person.

These issues are particularly salient in nursing because of the deep associations of the primary task with caring and nurturing. Yet many times patients are difficult, hateful, or demanding, thereby provoking aggressive feelings that should not be discharged in that relationship. Therefore, the emotions can easily be displaced onto others with whom we must collaborate. Furthermore, in work relationships we are often angry at someone who has considerable control over decisions we care about.

For example, harnessing our feelings of aggression against the pharmacy staff, who can easily retaliate by the way they deal with our future requests, can be problematic.

Anxieties About Control. Anxieties about control are particularly salient in the context of lateral relationships or cross-boundary relationships, in which the authority relationships are not given but must be negotiated (implicitly or explicitly) as the work gets done. The fear is of losing control, that both the substance and the process of the transaction will be dictated by the other person. The reactions to this fear are often to overstructure — to produce a tight agenda and clear procedure to stick with the facts, to avoid spontaneity. The paradox is that the more we control a situation, the less we are able to learn. We run the risk of being trapped in a self-fulfilling prophecy. Hospitals are replete with ambiguous relationship systems with bureaucratic hierarchies meshing with professional ad hocracies. Many relationships are negotiated (Strauss and others, 1964). Nurse-physician relationships particularly provoke anxieties over control. "Doctor's orders" belies the discretion that exists at the bedside.

Anxieties About Punishment. Anxieties about punishment are most evident in relationships upward or with those toward whom we have been aggressive. We fear that people above us or more powerful will punish us. Sometimes acting-out behavior is an unconscious way of provoking punishment from others because we think we "deserve" it. Often the fear of punishment leads to ingratiating behavior, wherein we seek out favors from those who are more powerful than we are. Hospitals are systems filled with anxiety about outcomes and the fear of mistakes (Bosk, 1979). These anxieties can often distort working relationships and result in defensive collaboration to ensure that the problems did not occur "on my watch."

These are some of the major anxieties that manifest themselves and unconsciously shape many of the dynamics in work systems. For example, an executive from a nonprofit organization boasted, "I would never hold a board meeting unless I could write the minutes in advance." His anxieties over losing control to a board whose role is to set policy and supervise his work result in no possibility of learning. In the long run he puts himself at risk with the very people he is so anxious to control.

These anxieties play a double role in distorting communications and working relationships. Directly, they alter the behavior and substance of communication so that, for example, bad news is not relayed up the chain of command or a situation is left uncorrected. Indirectly at another level, these anxieties also make it much less likely that the parties will ever directly discuss the difficulties in the relationship and thereby correct the misunderstandings. Paradoxically, those with whom we are having the most trouble may be the most powerful sources of information and learning. They may be our best collaborators.

Exchanging Role Perceptions

Exchanging role perceptions can be an effective way of resolving anxieties in work relationships. In this section I discuss some of the reflections that nursing leaders and their CEOs raised during a two-day session, called the "Executive Forum," which is part of the Johnson & Johnson–Wharton Fellows Program and is aimed at improving working alliances.

Participants were asked which aspects of their role they feel are invisible to the other and are underappreciated and which aspects are the most difficult to discuss. CEOs felt that the nurse executives are not sufficiently aware of how much time the board demands of them and the diversity they need to deal with in worrying about the big picture. They feel that their work and concern with the medical staff may not be sufficiently noticed by nursing. CEOs often feel that they are stereotyped by the nurse executives as being too bottom-line oriented, whereas in fact they are deeply concerned about quality. The nurse executive is often underaware of the real constraints that may shape some of the unpleasant decisions that the CEO and nurse executive must reach together.

The difficulties in the relationship as viewed by the CEOs make the following topics difficult to discuss openly:

1. Mutual expectations
2. Intangible aspects, such as other's style
3. The CEO's relationship to the medical staff
4. Resource allocation issues, because of the emotionality of
    the quality issues

In turn, the nurse executives feel that CEOs underappreciate nursing's role vis-à-vis professional practice issues, physician relationships, and patient relationships, especially given resource pressures. Even though the CEOs feel that they get drawn into the nurse-physician-administrator triangle, nurses feel that they cope with many physician conflicts that never get to administration. Nurses list issues similar to those of CEOs as difficult to discuss openly, but they add the gender issue. And unlike many of their peers in the top-management group, nurse executives must struggle with the joint role of advocating for a professional group and of being a top staff member with institutionwide concerns.

Overall, from the data produced by the discussions between the two groups, they are actually closer in understanding each other than they think. Each appears to have considerable empathy for the other's role and to know the pressures that each may think the other does not fully appreciate. This is the crux of the matter. Part of the reason there is some tension in this relationship is the role that third parties play in it. Despite the prevalence of dyadic relationships in organizations — for example, boss and subordinate — the triangle is really the building block of organizations (Gilmore, 1982b; Smith, 1984; Bowen, 1974). When a pair is under some stress, both individuals will often involve a third party as a strategy to deal with their conflict. Many variations are possible, but a classic pattern is for two elements to be intensely related, either positively or negatively, and a third party to be somewhat distant or uninvolved. The positions among the elements can change rapidly, with secrets and coalitions switching the different positions.

These dynamics are illustrated in nurse executives' key lateral relationship with the chief financial officer (CFO). Given the increased financial pressures, the link to the CFO is critical. Nurses often feel that the CFO is too influential and imagines that nursing can have more influence over the physicians (and costs) than is really the case. Nurses experience financial aspects that should be *constraints* on the best decision that can be made as too often the primary determinants of a decision. Role negotiations can be a powerful way to deepen the understanding in a critical work alliance (Harrison, 1976). The following list shows the major steps in the role negotiation process.

1. Introduction to role interdependence and importance of collaboration. Discuss process and establish ground rules.
2. Remind participants about characteristics of effective feedback. Messages should be:

   - hearable; the other should be able to tolerate being told about the behavior.
   - testable; the other should be able to test the meaning of the feedback by linking it to data that are accessible to observation — for example, "giving more lead time" can actually be measured, specific cases can be discussed, others can offer their perceptions, whereas "trusting me more" can be known only in the mind of the other.
   - actionable; the behavior should reference aspects of one's repertoire that can be modified.

3. Each member writes down three categories of behaviors he or she wants from each other in the group:

   - behaviors that you want *more of* from the other in order for you to be more effective in your role.
   - behaviors that you want *less of* in order for you to be more effective in your role.
   - behaviors that you value and want kept *the same* from the other because they help you to be effective in your role.

4. Exchange lists: Each individual has all lists about his or her behavior.

5. Each participant summarizes messages and posts those he or she is willing to work on.
6. Clarifying questions.
7. Identifying most negotiable items:

   - You willing.
   - Other willing.

8. Negotiate, contract, and document.

One nurse executive, in thinking through her relationship to her CFO, came up with the following role messages from her to the CFO:

More of

- Believing that I am also concerned about the bottom line and not always stereotyping me as only concerned with quality of care.
- Educating me and my people about financial management and the financial implications of decisions so that we become more competent over time to integrate these issues with our work.
- Complimenting me or people in my department when we deserve it.

Less of

- Chauvinism, assuming that because I am a woman and the department is composed mainly of women we are incompetent financially.
- Discounting of ideas and suggestions because they come from nursing.
- Feeling that he and finance are the only ones who care about the health of the total organization.

The same

- Humor.
- His commitment to the whole organization.

In addition to thinking of what she wanted to say to him, she thought of what he might want to say to her (in the format of role messages). She imagined his responses as follows:

More of

- Taking responsibility to meet the bottom line.
- Becoming articulate about the rationale and justification for your proposals. Do not presuppose that I understand the rationale for certain nursing practice issues (for example, the link between increased acuity and the staffing levels in the ICU).

Less of

- Battling over the budget; let's collaborate more.
- Reasons why you cannot meet the financial constraints; more problem solving to come up with responses that meet your needs and yet are within budget.
- Talking about increased acuity; I am sick to death of hearing how sick the patients are.
- Less going to the CEO to make special pleas for your concerns that upset the agreements I have worked out that balance competing demands across many departments.

The same

- Humor.
- Being a good manager of your department.

We can appreciate how useful this thinking process is to clarify relationships, even before we can get the other to participate. Just by thinking concretely about the other — what behaviors we want more of, less of, and the same of — we can prepare to capitalize on opportunities that might arise to give feedback to or influence the other through our own responses. Furthermore, thinking concretely about what the other might want from oneself is also powerful. Many times we begin to realize for the first time how little we really know about what the other wants. It can create the motivation either for risking actually having the conversation or for attending more carefully to the cues that are available.

When we discussed the nurse executive's role messages and the imagined set that the CFO would send, the following dilemma emerged. After a meeting she often felt so angry at his attitude and the pattern of behavior that she experienced in a meeting that she was unable to give him calm, rational feedback. Therefore, she either gave him the feedback while it was fresh and risked confirming her emotionality (in his eyes) or stored it up so that it was less linked to the actual behavior and ran the risk of his feeling sandbagged from being given feedback about old behavior. The overall stress surrounding the top team led to many fewer occasions when it felt safe to give feedback to top team members.

Note in the preceding example the distortions introduced by underlying anxieties about aggression, control, and punishment. The CFO is a critical figure for a nurse executive and can be a powerful enemy if she provokes him to anger. Furthermore, she often feels that the CEO favors finance in the process and timing of financial issues. They develop the forms, the timing, the process.

The process of role negotiation can be a powerful way to work privately on the critical relationships among the entire top team and downward with your own direct reports. First list the critical roles with which you feel interdependent. Then for each role, complete a role messages sheet, and next develop an imaginary set of role messages of what you think they want from you. Just from reflecting on this work, you can learn about the relationships — which ones were easy, which difficult to think about. For example, if you experience difficulty in imagining what the other wants from you, you may realize that you do not understand their point of view well enough to collaborate effectively with them.

Many times I have used this process as a third party by having each party give me role messages, after which I facilitate a meeting with both parties with the ground rule that I will not tell either party of the messages that the other wants to send. I discover that by thinking of the messages in advance, people are more willing to exchange the messages. At one meeting, one party began by saying, "I was thinking that there was nothing that I said to Tom that I would not be comfortable saying to you directly, and I am not sure why we have not found the time or the way to have this conversation before." Part of the process of giving concrete voice to one's thoughts is that they become less frightening. The primitive anxieties over aggression, control, and punishment become reduced by thinking specifically and sorting out which ones you feel comfortable communicating, and in what way, versus the ones that are too deep to address constructively. By writing them down, especially in the context of a strained relationship, you clarify your thinking, you metabolize and digest primitive ideas. You rehearse and practice so that the phrasing is the least likely to perpetuate the misunderstandings.

We often imagine that the most problematic relationships are upward and sideways because of the lower control and influence we have with these links. However, I often experience significant distortions in a downward direction. Developing role messages — especially what you think the other wants from you — can be a powerful way of preparing for a coaching conference or a performance appraisal. By thinking of how the other sees the issues you are better prepared to negotiate a win-win outcome (Fisher and Ury, 1981).

Quality of Group Thinking

When an issue creates stress for a group, frequently different roles become the container for the anxiety, or a pair of roles becomes stuck on the issue in a way that lets the group avoid the painful confrontation of the issue. A particular risk is for one role to become stereotyped as only thinking about one half of a problem and another about another aspect. As the previous example of role messages between a nurse executive and the CFO suggested, there is some evidence of a frequent pattern in which nursing is viewed as caring only about quality — because of associations with nurturing, bedside care, the alliance with the patient — and the CFO as advocating low cost. When roles become stereotyped, a particularly dysfunctional splitting can easily occur that distorts the true differences between them.

Assume a continuum of cost-quality trade-offs with a balanced position in the middle. Person A, who is arguing against someone whom she or he perceives as insensitive to the quality issue, B, may begin the conversation by overstating his or her true position in anticipation of the counterarguments of B. B, hearing the extreme statement, feeling that A has under-attended to the cost issues, responds by being a bit more extreme in advocating the other position. The dynamic continues with each getting more extreme and over time becoming less and less likely to discover that their true differences were significantly less than the expressed differences (see Figure 9.2).

Figure 9.2. Splitting Dynamics.

Expressed differences

True differences

QUALITY			COST
A's expressed position	A's true position	B's true position	B's expressed position

This is not just a political process and/or a negotiating ploy — that is, overstating your initial position in the hopes of getting a final compromise (split the difference) that is closer to your desired position. It has significant psychological dimensions for both the individuals and the groups in which this dynamic takes hold. One often unconsciously delegates some aspect of a problem to someone else so that one does not have to keep it in mind as part of thinking about the problem (Gilmore and Krantz, 1985). The effect of splitting, in this example cost from quality, is that one then does not have to wrestle with the painful choices that might be involved. At a group level, different people can become stuck in roles and their views only ritually attended to with no capacity to shape the debate.

The challenge to groups is to develop the ability to get all participants to think on *all* sides of a particular issue rather than play out a ritualized debate. An effective strategy is to make all participants speak to *both* sides, so that everyone is collaborating in thinking about the benefits and costs of a particular course of action.

One nurse executive commented on a pattern she experienced when the CFO obliterated the expression of others' points of view by dominating meetings and forcefully presenting finance's perspective on the issue. After a discussion of the situation, several points emerged. First, the CEO was clearly authorizing this behavior, either implicitly or explicitly, so that the relationship became at least a triangle. Second, another possibility was that the group colluded in such behavior because it was a way to channel the anxiety surrounding the difficult cost-quality trade-off issues that lay beneath the surface.

Responsibility Charting

I have looked at some of the interpersonal aspects of working alliances and the distortions that can impair the effectiveness of teams. Another source of variance in organizational performance stems from confusion over roles and responsibilities. *Responsibility charting* is a structured process that can enable the persons with interdependent roles to work through quickly and clearly how they will interrelate on key decisions (McCann and Gilmore, 1983; Gilmore, 1979, 1988). It is open ended and flexible and can easily be adapted and updated as new circumstances dictate, resulting in the clarity necessary for effective collaboration without the rigidity of bureaucracy that can stifle creativity.

Responsibility charting consists of three elements: a set of decisions, a set of participants or actors or roles, and a language for describing how any given participant will be involved in a specific decision. The first two elements form the horizontal and vertical axes of a matrix, and the types of participation fill in the cells. We have inherited from the military the classic distinction of staff and line when describing participation. Line roles are in the chain of command and accountable for a decision; staff roles are considered advisory. Modern business organizations and certainly health care settings have, however, a much richer repertoire in terms of how different people can collaborate on any given decision. I suggest beginning with the four different modes described below, although some organizations that have used this process have developed up to twelve different ways of participating. The codes for participation and their definitions are as follows:

A = approves, signs off, vetoes, is accountable for the quality of the decision.

R = responsible, expected to detect relevant trends in the area, shape the definition of the problem, assemble the necessary analytical information, and make a recommendation or suggest options. This role is accountable for errors of omission, if nothing happens when something should have been done, in addition to being accountable for the quality of a decision when the approving role accepts the recomendation.

C = must be consulted, not a veto role, not actively responsible, but has some information relevant to the decision or a critical role in implementation that makes her or his input valuable.

I = must be informed, prior to the decision being announced publicly, needs to know the results of the decision in order to do the work, but does not need to participate in the decision.

A Case Example: Working Through Product-Line Management. Imagine an organization that is growing rapidly in a state that has changed the rules of the game dramatically. The organization has three institutions with a fourth under construction, all operating under a corporate group. Each facility is headed by a vice president for operations and is held accountable for profitability, market share, and customer satisfaction. The strategy of product-line management has been adopted to focus on a few selected areas and to manage the interdependencies more effectively, but the result has been additional confusion rather than better coordination. It is in this situation that the top team employed responsibility charting as a way of working through the critical relationships.

After determining that the product-line concept was a major source of confusion, the group focused in on this area, each identifying critical decisions that were most unclear in terms

Figure 9.3. Responsibility Chart for Oncology Product Line.

Roles / Decisions	Vice president for operations	Product-line manager	Director of nursing	Chair of oncology	Administrator of surgery	Director of marketing	CFO	COO		
1. Strategic planning for oncology	A	R	C	A	C	C	C	A		
2. Marketing strategy	C	A	C	C		R				
3. Negotiating surgery slots for oncology	A	R		C	R					
4. Pricing the oncology products	A	C					R			
5. Resolving a nursing problem on an oncology unit	A	R	R							

of participation. Once they were listed, the group easily identified the actors or stakeholders in those decisions, resulting in the responsibility chart illustrated in Figure 9.3, with letters in the cells illustrating how one participant might have filled out the chart. The actors do not all have to be internal to the organization, although they are in this example. Outside stakeholders often play significant roles in key decisions.

Once the chart has been created, each participant ballots on how he or she sees the decisions actually being made. Staff or outside consultants then tabulate the information, or alternatively the group can work through the chart, discussing each decision in turn. Once the results are tabulated, the group has a clear map of the different perceptions surrounding the decisions. At this stage, the group works through the discrepancies. Some of the major implications of differences in how one sees one's own role and how others see it are indicated in Table 9.1.

Let us examine the discussion that ensued over one decision, that of setting price (decision 4 in Figure 9.3). In the initial balloting, of fourteen respondents, nine felt that the vice president for finance needed to approve price, and five thought he actually set the price. The role of the vice president for operations (VPO) was seen as predominantly advisory, except for the chief operating officer, who voted that the VPO needed to

Table 9.1. Analysis of Discrepancies.

You see your role as	Other sees it as	Consequence
A	R	Possible lack of action in this area, with you blaming others for not delivering when they in turn are looking to you.
R	A	You are given too little information, and you are involved later than you want in the decision process.
C	I	Other sees you as only needing to be informed.
I	C	Other will be drawing on your time, expecting input when you do not feel the need for involvement; possible delay.

approve price. His argument was, how could he hold the VPO accountable if she did not sign off on the price of key products? Note that this is not a majority rule process, but rather the perceptions are simply the catalyst to get richer thinking on why one configuration might be better than another. Most agreed that the product-line manager (PM) was responsible. The group then began to explore options for how these three roles (and levels) interacted on the pricing decision. The options are listed in Table 9.2. Note that without altering the formal table of organization, many choices are possible, each with different strengths and weaknesses. The group had a good discussion of this decision, weighing the need for finance's participation to integrate price setting with regulators' constraints and group sales against the desire to empower the product-line manager.

Table 9.2. Options for Setting Prices.

Option	PM	VPO	VPF	Comment
1	R	A	C	VPF as technical consultant
2	C	A	R	VPF as initiator, PM as consultant
3	R	A	A	Matrix, need dual approvals
4	R	C	A	VPF in control, VPO advising only
5	R	A	R	Collaborative, approval by VPO

Note that these differences do not determine who is in or out of a decision. A C role for finance may mean just as much time and effort as an A role, or even substantially more time. It is the nature of the involvement and the resultant patterns of accountability that shift.

When the group has worked through to a consensus or when the manager in charge of the process has heard the various arguments and reaches a decision, the chart can be a powerfully compact way to communicate the ground rules for decisions to key participants. In fact, an executive can use responsibility charting not as a diagnostic tool but simply to specify the way in which a key project will be accomplished (Gilmore and Peter, 1987).

Note the differences between a responsibility chart and a job description. For example, the product-line manager's job description might state "responsible for development of marketing strategy, overall management of the product line" without indicating that the former requires careful working relationships with corporate marketing and that the latter is under the direction of the VPO.

The process of working through a chart is valuable even if done by a single manager to explore the patterns of responsibility around a critical set of decisions. As each line is filled out, the manager can check the distribution of influence and pattern of participation for that decision.

1. Is there someone clearly in the lead (R) role? If there is more than one person, is it clear how they will work together? Are too many people in lead roles, as opposed to locating the authority in a single individual and letting others serve in other capacities?

2. What is the pattern of oversight? Are there multiple A's? Do all those people need to approve? Does each one add something to the review? Is there a risk that accountability will actually be reduced by each imagining that the other A role will review it carefully?

3. What is the pattern of consultation? Do all those people need to be involved? Are there people left out who might have valuable contributions or who might be angered by their lack of participation in ways that could affect implementation? Have the real costs and benefits of participation been carefully weighed? The following is a listing of the costs and benefits.

Costs	*Benefits*
• Lost time from delivering service or working on more important decisions	• New information about the issue
• Interruption and diffusion of focus from other tasks one is working on	• New perspectives on the issue

- Delay from waiting for different people to get to the issue

- Diffusion of accountability

- Information overload

- Potential cynicism from being "consulted" but not seeing the impact of one's ideas

- More ownership of the eventual decision and understanding of the reasons behind it, leading to more effective implementation

- Accountability: those responsible for an area should have some say in the decisions

4. Are the right people being informed?

5. Finally, one can look at the overall involvement in the decision and ask if more organizational resources (in terms of A's, R's, and C's) are being consumed, given the real importance of the decision in the overall scheme of things. Is the proposed pattern of responsibility an efficient one? The manager works through each decision, thinking about it horizontally, until the full set of decisions has been tentatively mapped out. Inevitably, as one works through the set, subsequent decisions have begun to be influenced by the initial patterns, putting responsibilities together that make sense and providing checks and balances. However, when the full chart has been worked through, the manager can now do some vertical scanning by each role to consider the following:

- Is any one role overloaded, carrying too much responsibility, needing to be involved in all discussions?
- Are there roles that are surprisingly underloaded, with few responsibilities, or are there line roles that only seem to have advisory (C) relationships to the decisions, which might suggest that they could be eliminated from participating in this project?
- Is the pattern of total influence by each role appropriate given the particular focus of the project?
- Does the type of participation fit with the skills and style of the role occupants?

Both the horizontal and vertical analyses can sometimes be helped by assigning weights to each type of participation (for example, $A = 4$, $R = 3$, $C = 2$) and doing column and row totals (Gilmore, 1982a). The row totals represent a crude estimate of the total amount of influence being expended on that decision. The column totals represent a crude score of the role importance for the set of decisions. Both can help the project manager think about the right pattern of investment of limited management time in getting a new venture successfully launched.

Once the manager has done these analyses and has readjusted the charts accordingly, he or she has a clear way of communicating to all the different players how they will relate to one another. In particular, if the process has not been used diagnostically with many people, rather than simply announcing it as a fact, it can be useful at this point to get some consultation on the proposed pattern, since other roles may see it differently. By sending the chart around with an adequate description of what the decisions are and what the different codes mean, the manager can get specific feedback from the people who will be participating in the project. Does anyone think his or her role, or the roles of others, should be different from what has been laid out? Note how nicely this works in communicating to a group of people how they will be interrelating without having to get them together in a face-to-face meeting (improbable, given the cast of characters and the different pressures on their time).

The Benefits of Responsibility Charting. Once people have given feedback and the charts have been modified accordingly, the group is then ready to go forward with a shared understanding of how they will be interrelating. What are some of the consequences of reaching such agreements?

1. Increased accountability results. People have in effect signed on to participate in specific ways and are in a much more powerful position to hold one another accountable. Feedback upward in an organization is more likely to occur when the criteria are clear and there has been prior agreement.

Furthermore, given the pressure for entrepreneurial activity, responsibility charting clearly locates the R role and can therefore hold people accountable for errors of omission, something that bureaucracies find very difficult to do. Table 9.3 shows the relationship of the participation codes to the different types of accountability.

Table 9.3. Different Types of Accountability.

Two Major Types of Error:
 OMISSION: No action when there should have been
 COMMISSION: Mistakes, poor decisions

Relationship to Decision	Consequence — Accountable for:
A	Error of Commission
R	Commission (if advice followed) and Omission (if failure to initiate action) (accountable for ensuring that those with C role are consulted)
C	Accuracy of Advice (but even if followed no accountability for decisions)
I	No Accountability for Decision (could be accountable for failure to act on decision if properly informed)

2. Delegations are clarified. Most of the writing on delegation assumes that it occurs from superiors to subordinates, so that the nature of the relationships is clear and only the task must be mutually agreed on. In actual fact, many delegations take place horizontally, upward, and so on, and in these cases both the substance and the nature of the relationship must be clear. Table 9.4 shows the relationships of different types of delegation and the participation codes.

3. People know their jobs in the context of other people's jobs. Members of well-run organizations, like great basketball teams, not only know their own assignments but also know those of others, so that they instinctively know when to collaborate with other members of the team. Job descriptions are like position descriptions in a sport. They say what the

Table 9.4. Delegation and Responsibility Charting.

Delegation	Delegatee	Meaning
A	R	Staff the decision, get the necessary facts, present the options, make a recommendation, and bring it to me for final review.
C	A/R	This is your decision, but consult with me to get my views. You are not bound by my advice; you are accountable for the decision.
A/R	C	Let me keep the decision and manage the fact finding and analysis of options, but give me your best thinking.
I	A/R	This is your decision; merely inform me of the outcome.

role does but do not show how it links with others to accomplish results. In a sense, responsibility charting is like a play book that shows how different roles collaborate to achieve goals.

4. Because responsibility agreements are so specific, they are easily updated and modified. They address the specific issue at hand, but they can also serve as a precedent for similar decisions. Responsibility agreements help the organization begin to develop an evolving pattern of interrelating without having to specify it in advance via some grand reorganization scheme or promulgated policies.

5. Time expectations can be established for each step and for the project. Delays in one can affect the others, and adjustments are more easily made when those with oversight responsibility can clearly see the patterns of interdependency.

6. The overall responsibility chart gives the patterns for the major decisions. When each department gets this guidance, the very same process is useful to examine at a finer grain how that unit will get its part of the total job done. This gives the process a zoom-lens quality, in which one can choose the appropriate degree of resolution depending on the stage of the project.

Implementation Issues

In the previous sections, I have introduced the structured processes of role negotiation and responsibility charting. Both are vehicles for stepping back from the direct relationship to reflect on it and to check for distortions that may be interfering with work. In this type of work, there are two dimensions that are significant: one's own openness to change and the degree of "publicness" of one's testing or inquiring about the issues. Table 9.5 illustrates the interactions of these two dimensions. If one is

Table 9.5. Testing Strategies for Working Through Differences.

| | | Testing | |
		Private	Public
Attitude Toward Change	Closed	Compatible in that not opening up the issue is likely to keep the status quo.	Can be risky to open areas in which you are closed to change.
	Open	Change can only be as effective as the accuracy of your private diagnosis. You may miss opportunities because of untested assumptions that are not true. Danger of self-fulfilling prophecies.	High-learning mode, get feedback on your views and can change accordingly.

not open to changing one's own behavior, then the most appropriate strategy is to test privately (upper left in the table). Once one is open to change, only to test one's hunches privately exposes one to the risk of self-fulfilling prophesies. The high-learning quadrant is both to be open to change and to test publicly. For many the dilemma is that although one feels ready to discuss critical relationship issues, the key other (often a powerful peer or superior) is not perceived to be ready. There are risks to opening discussions of certain issues, and one clearly needs to be selective. Paradoxically, by being specific about which issues one is closed to, one often gains credibility in discussions about those one is genuinely open to. People are understandably suspicious in a situation in which no limits have been set and may mistake it for not caring or taking the discussion lightly. If significant issues that you are known to care about are raised, people will often respond to the risks you have taken by collaborating in genuine ways. The following list offers a number of questions that can be useful in thinking through a poorly functioning working alliance.

1. How far are the issues role related rather than personal (for example, goes with territory)? Inventory the differences on either side of the boundary in terms of time horizon, goals, motivation, values, and so on. Which differences seem most significant?

2. What can be learned from reflecting on the history of the relationship? Has it ever been significantly better? Or worse? What factors seem linked to changes in the relationship?

3. What are the task and/or performance costs to the lack of development in the relationship? What would be the benefits of significant improvement, and how would they be distributed among the parties?

4. Often what appear as two-person issues are triangular in their underlying structure. Who are potential third parties to the relationship you are looking at, and how might they be contributing? What are the usual alliances? Are there indirect strategies that might improve the relationship? Is the relationship significantly different when others are present?

5. Imagine an exchange of role messages with this person. What specific behaviors would you want more of, less of, and the same of from them? What do you think they would want from you?

6. How clear are your respective responsibilities? Is it clear who has the lead on which issues, who must be consulted, who has ultimate authority?

7. Imagine communicating your concerns to this person with no interpersonal inhibitions. What are the main outlines

of what you want to say? Contrast that with what you do communicate. What aspects are difficult to discuss? Why? What might be the risks?

8. What forums do you have for reflecting on and discussing the relationship (as opposed to transacting business)? Could any be created? Are there intermediators who could play facilitative roles?

Responsibility charting is a clarifying process and as such is not neutral with respect to the politics of an organization. Politics in a complex medical center organization includes conflict, consensus building, and bargaining among people with diverse interests and unequal influence. Organizational behavior emerges from intricate, subtle, simultaneous, and overlapping games among "players" located in positions in the hierarchy. Regular channels structure the game; deadlines force issues to the attention of incredibly busy people. The decisions and sequence of actions are explained in terms of agreements among players with separate judgments and shared power in the organization.

Often certain roles and people have a vested interest in ambiguity because they are able to use it as a source of influence (Pfeffer and Salancik, 1977), and the use of these tools will therefore require careful introduction. Specifying the patterns of participation does not mean that politics has been eliminated from the decision process. To the contrary, we would argue that it enables sharper substantive disagreements with a shared understanding of the process.

The use of the structured technique of responsibility charting can be a powerful tool to open up the decision-making process. It frames the questions "What is the issue?" and "What must be done?" It has the potential to improve the planning process and to help the organization avoid costly mistakes and errors of omission. Players who supported the decision will work to see it implemented. Retrospectively it enables the organization to examine why a project succeeded or failed and to learn from the experience.

Many times people who are unhappy with a particular outcome say that they do not so much mind the result as object to the process. This is most often a tactic to delay a decision. They focus on the process because they think that they have a better chance of thwarting the decision on procedural than on substantive grounds. Signing off on the patterns of participation can powerfully reduce the potential after-the-fact procedural challenges to the outcome.

The most difficult aspect of implementation is to build within a scattered group sufficient understanding of the process, especially the definitions of the decisions and the types of participation. If people have different understandings of the decisions (for example, "When you said hiring, I was thinking of the paperwork, and you were thinking of the interviewing"), or assign different meanings to the key codes (A, R, C, I), then the process will not introduce any consistency into the actual behavior because people will not be aware of what they are agreeing to.

Clearly the most powerful way to build understanding is to introduce the process via some management development program so that it becomes part of the organization's culture. Alternatively, one can begin within one's own unit, and only slowly start to use it with one or two other groups so that over time a wider awareness exists as regards its potential. For it to be really useful in disciplining multiunit agreements, ultimately the top leadership must become comfortable with the process. Top leaders often benefit from ambiguity because it forces more of the choices back to their offices. As the challenges to the institution mount, therefore, it becomes even more important for top leaders to be able to make the guiding policy choices and then delegate them clearly to others so that their own time is freed up to focus on the strategic choices facing their institutions.

Conclusion

Beneath the strategic challenges that health care organizations are experiencing are critical working relationships. Underlying working alliances are many potential anxieties that can block effective communication. The clarity of thinking with which a group can address new challenges will be shaped by the quality of working alliances and by the awareness within the group of the distortions that can intrude. The following strategies can keep critical working alliances in three directions in good repair:

1. The parties at the top of complex, fast-changing organizations need to find the time to reflect on roles and relationships and how strategic challenges are reshaping them. There is a major difference between actually transacting business and reflecting on the transacting of business. Many people who work together every day never have direct conversation that reflects on their patterns of interaction (although they may have complained frequently to a friend or spouse or colleague). People need to take greater risks in raising these issues *because* the stakes are high. They need to think more about the distortions they feel when having these conversations upward and to find more effective ways to help their subordinates give them better feedback. Too often we begin with what we want to tell someone else as opposed to working on our inquiry skills to import new perspectives that might have implications for our behavior.

2. Often retreats are powerful vehicles for reflection on working relationships while also thinking about long-range substantive issues. I am always struck by people's ability to get away for conferences and training events, but too often they do not get the real group of people that they must collaborate with daily into similarly protected settings for sustained discussions. Particularly when the retreats break the normal daily routines and work into the evening or integrate recreation and work, new understandings can result. Third-party facilitation can sometimes be useful in helping a group to gain perspective on itself or to see aspects of its own group process that live beneath awareness (Hirschhorn, 1990).

3. Structured tools such as responsibility charting and role negotiation can be powerful ways to contain the anxiety engendered by direct discussion of relationship issues. Both are clearly linked to the work at hand and avoid purely interpersonal issues. Both offer initial individual reflection,

which then coalesces and reaches out to explore group-level patterns. These tools are artificial, but that weakness is also their strength in that they interfere with the standard operating procedures that guide everyday behaviors and allow people to see the broader patterns.

4. Spend time thinking about and working on those relationships that are dysfunctional. We often flee from the intensity of difficult relationships. Do not let yourself simply label the problem as residing in the other's personality.

5. On new projects, anticipate the relationship issues and invest in some early discussions of the critical issues, how the project might fail, who will play what roles. Role negotiating and responsibility charting are powerful ways to help a newly formed team develop realistic expectations of one another before people become disappointed on the basis of perceptions and hopes that were never shared.

The rapid rate of change is creating greater stress for health care organizations and increasing both the difficulties of collaborating and the imperatives of doing so. The investment by the top group in the tools of role negotiation and responsibility charting and in creating greater shared awareness of dilemmas surrounding working alliances can greatly enhance the capacity of an organization to adapt and cope with unfolding strategic challenges.

References

Bosk, C. *Forgive and Remember: Managing Medical Failure.* Chicago: University of Chicago Press, 1979.

Bowen, M. "Bowen on Triangles—March 1974 Workshop Park 1." *The Family,* 1974, *2* (1), 45–48.

Fisher, R., and Ury, W. *Getting to Yes: Negotiating Agreement Without Giving In.* Boston: Houghton Mifflin, 1981.

Gilmore, T. N. "Managing Collaborative Relationships in Complex Organizations." *Administration in Social Work,* 1979, *3* (2), 167–180.

Gilmore, T. N. "Leadership and Boundary Management." *Journal of Applied Behavioral Science,* 1982a, *18* (3), 343–356.

Gilmore, T. N. "A Triangular Framework: Leadership and Followship." In R. Sagar and K. Wiseman (eds.), *Understanding Organizations: Applications of Bowen Family Systems Theory.* Washington, D.C.: Family Center, Georgetown University, 1982b.

Gilmore, T. N. *Making a Leadership Change: How Organizations and Leaders Can Handle Leadership Transitions Successfully.* San Francisco: Jossey-Bass, 1988.

Gilmore, T. N., and Krantz, J. "Projective Identification in the Consulting Relationship: Exploring the Unconscious Dimensions of a Client System." *Human Relations,* 1985, *38* (12), 1159–1177.

Gilmore, T. N., and Peter, M. A. "Managing Complexity in Health Care Settings." *Journal of Nursing Administration,* 1987, *17* (1), 11–17.

Harrison, R. "Role Negotiation: A Tough-Minded Approach to Team Development." *Social Technology of Organization Development.* La Jolla, Calif.: University Associates, 1976.

Hirschhorn, L. *Managing in the New Team Environment.* Reading, Mass.: Addison-Wesley, 1990.

McCann, J. E., and Gilmore, T. N. "Diagnosing Organizational Decision Making Through Responsibility Charting." *Sloan Management Review,* 1983, *29* (2), 3–15.

Peters, T. J., and Austin, N. *A Passion for Excellence.* New York: Random House, 1985.

Peters, T. J., and Waterman, R. H. *In Search of Excellence: Lessons from America's Best Run Companies.* New York: Harper & Row, 1982.

Pfeffer, J., and Salancik, G. R. "Organizational Design: The Case for a Coalitional Model of Organization." *Organizational Dynamics,* 1977, *6,* 15–29.

Segal, J. *Phantasy in Everyday Life: A Psychoanalytical Approach to Understanding Ourselves.* Harmondsworth, England: Penguin Books, 1985.

Smith, K. K. "Towards a Conception of Organizational Currents." *Group and Organizational Studies,* 1984, *9* (2), 285–312.

Strauss, A., and others. *Psychiatric Ideologies.* Glencoe, Ill.: Free Press, 1964.

Weick, K. E. "Educational Organizations as Loosely-Coupled Systems." *Administrative Science Quarterly,* 1976, *21,* 1–19.

CHAPTER 10

Negotiation
as Problem Solving

Gregory P. Shea

Consider: You walk into an encounter thinking, "This is a bargaining session." Think of all that accompanies that assumption: all the images, postures struck, games played, demands issued, and ultimatums delivered.

Now consider this. You walk into an encounter thinking, "This is a problem-solving session." Think of what accompanies that assumption: working to define the problem accurately, getting all relevant data on the table, brainstorming alternatives, sorting through options, and specifying next steps.

Consider the differences between these encounters, in terms both of how you approach what happens *and* of what actually happens. These differences stem from how the encounters are defined, namely, as problem-solving sessions or as bargaining sessions. That reorientation is as powerful as it is basic and therefore difficult. That reorientation is the focus of this chapter.

Procedure

When we receive information out of context, we have a hard time retaining it. The problem occurs because we do not know

Note: I wish to thank all the participants in the Leonard Davis Institute and Johnson & Johnson workshops for helping me to develop my thinking about negotiation as problem solving. And more specifically, I am indebted to the Harvard Negotiation Project for shaping the thinking in the sections titled "A Word About Mindsets" and "Hard Problem Solving: Underpinnings and Techniques."

why we are receiving the information. We do not see how it fits into our world or, more to the point, what difference knowing it will make — what use it might serve — and hence we discard it. We are deluged with information, so we attend to what appears useful.

Too often management seminars or workshops amount to information received out of context. The participants are left to forge a link between the subject matter and the specifics of their world, including their experiences to date and upcoming issues. In one sense, it is fair that the work of forging is left to participants. After all, detailed customization should be what consulting is all about, not stand-up workshops. Nonetheless, the work of forging can begin in seminars and workshops. Their structure, for example, can facilitate linking previous experience and forthcoming challenges to a given workshop.

That said, it is time to pause and look backward. Think back through your experiences both at work and outside of work. Think about conflict situations in which you have been involved. Think of the ones in which your actions affected the outcome — for better or for worse. Do *not* revisit those situations that were apparently fated for successful resolution or for bitter endings. Concentrate only on conflictual situations whose resolution in retrospect you believe you affected. Select one such situation that you feel you handled well and one that you feel you handled badly. Jot down a few notes about each situation, the kind of notes that a reporter might take: who was involved, what the key events were and when they occurred, where the action transpired, and how the saga unfolded. (Set aside the "Why did it happen as it happened?" question for the moment.) A sketch is what you are after, not a tome. Be brief, yet jot enough down so that you are back in touch with what happened in each case. One test of whether or not you have made contact with your past is whether or not you arrive at the point of feeling something about the situation. Usually, conflict situations are aswirl with emotions, and truly revisiting them involves tapping emotional as well as intellectual memory.

Next, ask yourself these questions about the two situations:

1. Specifically, how could you tell that the situation was (was not) handled well?

2. What did *you* do?
3. What was the impact of what you did?
4. What was the consequence of the situation turning out the way it did?
5. If you could change anything about what *you* did, then what would you change?

Examine the notes that you have made. One of the key aspects of many conflict situations is how we handle the "negotiation." There is disagreement about what should happen next — our behavior and that of the other(s) involved — and you have to negotiate, or problem-solve, a way out. Take a look at what *you* did differently in the two situations. Perhaps talk to a friend about the two situations. A few more questions might help in comparing the two situations: Did you become locked into a position? How were emotions such as anger handled? How well did you listen, that is, did you learn anything about the situation while you were in it? Did you get *discussed,* not just said, what you wanted discussed? Was there a delivery problem, that is, did one or more of the parties subsequently fail to deliver what they promised to deliver?

The point here has been to open your files. Keep them open as we progress, and think about both the tactics you use when negotiating and the context that you bring to negotiation, that is, how you understand what happens and why *you* act as you do.

A Word About Mindsets

What would a good negotiation look like? How would we know one if we saw one? Here are some criteria (Fisher and Ury, 1981):

1. If an agreement was possible, an inspired agreement was reached, namely, everyone "won" something of value.
2. The word *streamlined* characterizes the process as a whole, from the first indication that a potential conflict or problem existed through to and including implementation and monitoring of an agreed-on solution.

3. The relations among the negotiators were better after the process was completed than before it began.

    This definition of good negotiation is not well served by walking into a room with a mind filled with images of traditional hard bargaining. Such images include bidding ridiculously high or low — frequently with derision thrown in for good measure, grudging concessions of minuscule proportion, conscious deception about facts *and* feelings, and no attempt to understand the other side's position, let alone problem.

    Hard bargaining has its place. It may fit if you do not really need what you are bargaining over or if you might not need the person with whom you are bargaining — now or in the future. Hard bargaining may fit when the situation really entails a single win-lose issue. (Beware: We often prematurely code issues as single win-lose issues, and once we act accordingly it is at best a difficult road back to problem solving.) Hard bargaining may also fit if your reputation is *not* at stake (this issue will be discussed later).

    However, even if traditional hard bargaining appears to fit, recognize that it tends to be inefficient; posturing both takes time itself and robs time from problem solving. Traditional hard bargaining also makes it decidedly less likely that creative solutions will emerge, because creativity flourishes best in supportive, non-evaluative settings. In addition, traditional hard bargaining usually disfigures relationships; unions and management seldom recover from strident negotiations over two- or three-year contracts before the time comes to negotiate the next contract, and divorce struggles rarely serve as the link between marriage and friendship.

    As for reputation, traditional hard bargaining takes a special toll. The hard bargainer, as defined here, develops a reputation as a rough opponent. Oddly enough, the hard bargainer also develops a reputation as someone not to be taken seriously, at least not at first. Word goes out that initial bargaining sessions with him or her are mere formalities stuffed with posturing. The hard bargainer pays a heavy price for the reputation, namely, time. His or her bargaining will take longer, in part because others become resigned to its taking longer.

A workable alternative to traditional hard bargaining exists: principled negotiation. Principled negotiation is most appropriate when the possibility of an inspired outcome exists, when the issues that could appear on the negotiating table are joint and involve multiple related questions and people (the more moving parts, the greater the likelihood of a win-win match occurring), and when the relationship among the negotiators may continue after the negotiations.

Principled negotiation is *not* soft negotiation; it is not sacrifice in the hope of receiving either mercy or goodwill. It is perhaps best differentiated from traditional hard bargaining by being defined as hard problem solving. The following section details the theory and practice of principled negotiation.

Hard Problem Solving: Underpinnings and Technique

Any hard problem solving involves six steps:

1. *Identification.* Something happens to suggest that a problem exists. A blip appears on a monitor, a memo arrives, a hallway conversation occurs.
2. *Clarification.* Does a problem actually exist? What is the *real* problem? Is what we originally identified as the problem really the problem or a symptom of something else?
3. *Alternative Generation.* Possible solutions to the clarified problem are listed. Brainstorming or blue-skying best fits here.
4. *Selection.* The criteria for determining the best alternative are selected, and those criteria are applied to the alternatives generated.
5. *Implementation.* This means doing it — putting the selected alternative in place.
6. *Feedback.* This involves checking to see if the problem, as identified and as clarified, goes away and stays away.

Figure 10.1 charts these basic problem-solving steps. Note the vertical line dividing the steps in half. Look at the steps to the left of the line and those to the right and ask yourself what makes the two sides of the line different.

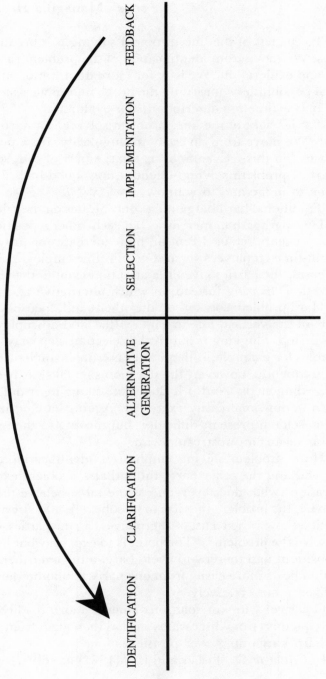

Figure 10.1. Six Problem-Solving Steps.

To the left of the line, problem solving is a broadening process. We move from identification of the problem to elaboration and exploration. We look for more information and additional possibilities concerning the problem or issues *and* solutions. It is a time for description, not evaluation.

To the right of the line, problem solving is a narrowing process. We move from diversity to singularity, from possible actions to "do this." Evaluation is a large part of the work of this part of problem solving — right/wrong, good/bad. This is the time to judge and to winnow.

Traditional hard bargaining concentrates on the selection step. Two parties hammer away at each other's positions — granting 5-cent- versus 3-cent-an-hour increases or providing three full-time employees versus one full-time employee. In too many cases, the parties give little attention even to the criteria for selection, fixating instead on which alternative to choose.

Hard problem solving, on the other hand, focuses on the left side of the vertical line in Figure 10.1 and downplays the selection step. Slugging it out in the selection step may prove inevitable, for example, if the matter is truly a single win-lose issue. Frequently, however, the selection step falls easily out of the preceding steps. And if it does not? Slugging it out is always an option, one easily exercised. Again, moving in that direction seldom presents difficulty, but moving in the reverse direction means an upstream swim.

Hard problem solving emphasizes identification (what makes you and the other party think that a problem exists?), clarification (what does everyone at the table believe the real issue to be, the problem that has to be solved?), and alternative generation (how varied a list of alternatives can the parties generate to solve the problem?). The point is to explore what lies behind positions and thereby to avoid bargaining over them. Information flows more easily from one party to another and can be utilized more creatively.

Creative, win-win solutions emerge more readily (and more frequently) from discussions such as these than from traditional hard bargaining over positions.

In *Getting to Yes,* Fisher and Ury (1981) use different lan-

guage to make similar points. (A more academic treatment of
the topic appears in Raiffa, 1982.) Fisher and Ury present four
principles:

1. Separate the people from the problem.
2. Focus on interests, not positions.
3. Invent options for mutual gain.
4. Insist on objective criteria.

Points 2 and 3 represent what we have just discussed,
namely, that what lies behind positions — interests — matters most
and that options for mutual gain need inventing; they do not
just happen. Point 4, insisting on objective criteria, amounts
to hard problem solving about a key part of the right side of
the vertical line in Figure 10.1: selecting the criteria for sorting
through alternatives generated. Fisher and Ury stress that the
criteria should be objective. The criteria might draw on standards (for example, the price of service provided will be 10 percent below market price) or procedure (for instance, turning
the selection of a work site over to a mutually agreed-on third
party). Regardless, the criteria should be clearly objective and
therefore readily applicable. Point 1, separating the people from
the problem, facilitates the entire hard-problem-solving process.
Both the problems and the relationships merit attention, separate
and distinct attention. Our tendency to express our frustration
with problems, for example, by insulting the other party, is both
understandable and self-destructive in that it impedes the problem-solving process. Similarly, expressing frustration with the
other party's personal style by obstructing problem solving con-
founds the matter and helps no one.

If the problem is the issue, then deal with it. If the person is the issue, then deal with him or her. For example, a cheap
shot taken at you or your staff requires that one form of hard
problem solving stops and another begins, namely, discussion
of the rules of the game. The same hard-problem-solving format applies to the new discussion, the "how we will bargain"
discussion, as applied to the main bargaining discussion: Identify the problem, clarify it, generate alternatives, select one, im-

plement it, and collect feedback. Hard problem solving fits most issues, including the issue of how to hard-problem-solve.

Fisher and Ury offer practical advice on how to put principled negotiation into practice, including chapters headed "What If They Are More Powerful?", "What If They Won't Play?", and "What If They Use Dirty Tricks?". One other aspect of their approach warrants attention here, namely, "Best Alternative to a Negotiated Agreement," or BATNA. The advice behind BATNA is straightforward and hard nosed: Know what your best alternative will be if negotiations fail. Restated, the purpose of hard problem solving or principled negotiation is to produce a better alternative than you already have. The purpose is *not* to produce *an* agreement. Preparing for principled negotiation consequently entails careful exploration of alternatives, however uninteresting or even unattractive they may initially seem. Having alternatives to a negotiated agreement allows you to know a bad deal when you see one (it is worse than what you could otherwise get) and to avoid wasting time considering offers amounting to less than your BATNA. Again, hard problem solving is not *soft* bargaining any more than it is traditional hard bargaining.

Another major difference between hard problem solving and soft bargaining is that hard problem solving includes verification about how the parties will know that the agreement works. Successful arms treaties and interdepartmental scheduling accords include specific, objective, measurable, mutually agreed-on gauges. The mere existence of the gauges ensures at least two desirable ends: First, discussion of how the parties can check on each other occurs, thereby making them more aware of the realities of how the agreement can work and of the ongoing nature of this agreement as well as of their relationship. Second, that discussion makes a follow-up discussion more likely, thereby increasing the chances that the agreement will live. That discussion does not, of course, ensure compliance. But it changes the odds in a desired fashion.

Hard problem solving is a place to start negotiations and a place to return to should you feel that your discussions are bogged down in step 4 (selection), that is, positional bargaining. Using it requires an overall appreciation of the process as well as a commitment to specific actions. Here is a list of those actions, both internal to one's self and involving other parties. The actions appear in a likely order of occurrence.

1. Know your BATNA.
2. Be willing to own 51 percent of the responsibility for effective communications.
3. Remember
   - our inherent tendency to blame problems on other people (as opposed to the situation in which they found themselves).
   - you need this person tomorrow.
   - replacing this person will cost you money.
4. Remain calm and make sure that the discussion is private.
5. Take the time necessary for a full discussion of the situation.
6. Move through the problem-solving steps.
7. Encourage the other person to elaborate his or her point of view.
8. Listen carefully to what the other person says and state your understanding of it.
9. State your opinion calmly and clearly and ask the other person to state his or her understanding of your point of view.
10. Concentrate on specific events or actions.
11. If an assumption or inference appears, check its validity.
12. Attempt to reach agreement, where possible, on what happened.
13. Clarify disagreements in as specific terms as possible.
14. Exchange ideas on what to do next about what was agreed on.
15. Exchange ideas on what to do next about what was not agreed on.
16. Draft a follow-up plan.
17. Monitor implementations of the plan.

When and with Whom to Use What You Now Know

Earlier, we discussed briefly the advantages of hard problem solving. At that time, we addressed the question of its most appropriate and timely use. Let us return to that question now, equipped with a better understanding of hard problem solving, and answer it in more detail. Richard Walton (1987, p. 155) presents four elements of conflict episodes: "issues, triggering events, conflict or conflict-resolving acts of the principals, and their consequences." Walton is speaking of interpersonal conflict, but his elements appear suited to help answer the more general question of when to use hard problem solving, namely, during any element of conflict episodes. (Often, of course, distinguishing between interpersonal, group, and systemic conflict carries important theoretical and practical implications. A detailed treatment appears in Shea, 1980.) Hard problem solving fits sorting through underlying issues, events that brought them to the surface, actions taken in light of the issues (and in reaction to events), and the residue of those actions.

Of central importance here is the concept of retreating from positions. A position or a demand flows easily when conflict occurs, especially when the conflict has a past history. A position taken because of the consequence of an action, the fact of the action, an event that brings up an issue (or brings it up again), or the very existence of an issue is still a position taken. The challenge remains to resist the temptation to engage in hard or positional bargaining and, failing that, to regroup and move to the left side of the vertical line in Figure 10.1 as quickly as possible. Doing so can prove useful in hard problem solving about, say, the consequences of an action, and it facilitates more fundamental problem solving, that is, moving from consequences toward underlying issues. In short, then, hard problem solving has general applicability to different stages or elements of conflict.

Answering the question of with whom to use hard problem solving requires a preliminary word about stakeholders. The concept of stakeholders has received attention of late (Freeman, 1984). The key premise for our purposes is that for any job a great number of individuals and groups exist that believe or that could believe at any time that they have a vested interest or a stake in how that job is performed. Stakeholders can materialize from both inside and outside your work area, department, and organization.

One way to define a job is in terms of its stakeholders, since performing a job necessarily entails successfully managing relations with those individuals and groups that believe they deserve a say in how that job is performed. The problem in successfully managing stakeholders has at least three dimensions. First, stakeholders are numerous. If you doubt this, then take out a sheet of paper and start listing the individuals and groups (including agencies) that believe (*they* believe) that they have a stake in how you do your job. Second, stakeholder objectives and values differ and frequently are in conflict. Third, each stakeholder comes fully equipped with his or her or their own set of stakeholders, who need managing in turn. That too should be part of hard problem solving: helping decide how to handle the key stakeholders that each negotiator needs to handle. Otherwise, the deal will have the shortest of lives.

Each manager needs to decide how much time to spend with which stakeholders and how to handle the time spent, especially when conflict exists. A brief consideration of this issue will help to answer the question of with whom to hard-problem-solve. For starters, those stakeholders who can have the greatest impact on whatever issue or problem is at hand merit the most attention. To help people discriminate, Block (1987) considers creating and implementing a vision. In the process, he presents a matrix categorizing how people will react to your vision (Figure 10.2). If we take the liberty of substituting issue or action for vision and stakeholder for people, then we can more readily apply Block's words (1987, p. 151) to help us decide how to spend what time with whom in the service of hard problem solving: Looking at the choices we have in building support, our goal is to move people toward the upper-right-hand quadrant of the matrix in the figure—to increase trust and agreement. It makes sense to spend most of our time with current allies and to seek new ones. A well-articulated vision statement and authentic behavior are the best ways to find the support. Our second level of energy goes to our opponents. They teach us about the marketplace for our ideas and help us perform more effectively. They also tend to speak well of us when we are not in the room. People will listen to them because it is known that our opponents do not agree with us on everything. The third order of priority is bedfellows. We want their support, and it takes rather persistent contact to maintain a fragile level of trust. Fence sitters become a passing fancy because they are finally going to take a position based on breezes outside their control. As for adversaries, two more meetings are all that are required: one meeting to try to negotiate trust or agreement one more time, then one to confess and say goodbye. If, despite all this eloquent prose, you choose to keep on trying to convert or destroy your adversaries, your next book should be *Winning Through Intimidation, or You Are What You Eat. Authentic behavior* for Block includes large amounts of what we have termed hard problem solving. Briefly stated, hard problem solving fits regardless of the stakeholder's orientation; how much time you wish to spend with even a key stakeholder is a separate matter.

Figure 10.2. Classifying Stakeholders: Take 1.

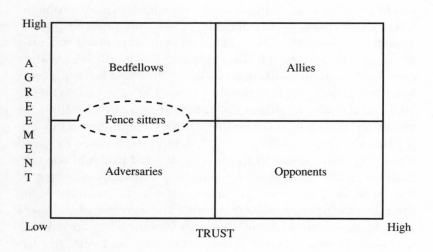

Source: Block, P. *The Empowered Manager: Positive Political Skills at Work.* San Francisco: Jossey-Bass, 1987, p. 132. Reproduced with permission.

And what if you *must* negotiate with an especially un-cooperative stakeholder? Fisher and Ury stress the value of BATNA, the power of trying to problem-solve with the stake-holder about the manner of negotiation, and separating the peo-ple from the problem. Another approach involves another matrix, one developed by John Eldred of the Wharton School of the University of Pennsylvania.

The basis of this matrix is that negotiators vary markedly in their underlying motivation and in their ability to hard-problem-solve. Either motivation or ability can hamper effec-tive negotiation, and knowing which it is makes all the differ-ence in how you try to move your partner or partners toward hard problem solving. Obviously, you hard-problem-solve with someone both competent to and willing to hard-problem-solve. If, however, your partner possesses the competence and lacks the motivation, then you had best spend your time working on how to induce your partner to use his or her skills. Perhaps in-centives for such involvement exist—your partner may be sim-ply unaware of them—in which case you have only to demon-strate that the incentives exist. Perhaps incentives do not exist. That is where hard problem solving begins: in identifying and securing the necessary incentives.

A highly motivated but incompetent partner needs edu-cation. The bargaining "partner" needs assistance in learning a new set of rules for negotiation. This partner may appear simi-lar to a partner needing greater inducements (that is, he or she is not actively contributing to hard problem solving), but add-ing inducements in this case or even problem solving about how to secure more inducements will only waste resources—especially time—and will probably increase everyone's frustration. Early on, discussion should focus on how best to equip the partner with the skills necessary for him or her to negotiate in the way that you both want to negotiate. Here is a case in which atten-dance by one or more of the parties at a brief workshop might do wonders. Finally, if the stakeholder has low competence and low motivation, then wait and see. Keep an eye out for signs of change (for example, use hard problem solving when you *have* to deal with this partner and note what happens), and in the meantime concentrate on improving your BATNA. (Figure 10.3 presents a summary of Eldred's matrix.)

Again, hard problem solving fits regardless of the stakeholder. Accurate diagnosis of the stakeholder informs you, however, about the advisability of the appropriateness of different types of "preparatory" work.

Whom to Try This Out on First

Give yourself a break. Give the method of hard problem solving a chance. Think small. Think necessary, even unavoidable. Think success.

Figure 10.3. Classifying Stakeholders: Take 2.

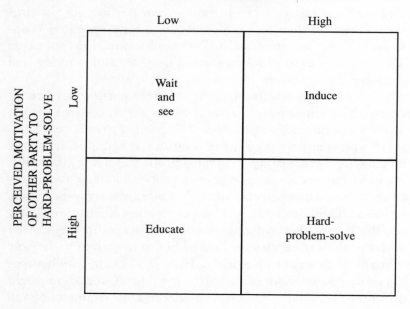

PERCEIVED COMPLIANCE OF OTHER
PARTY TO HARD-PROBLEM-SOLVE

	Low	High
Low	Wait and see	Induce
High	Educate	Hard-problem-solve

(PERCEIVED MOTIVATION OF OTHER PARTY TO HARD-PROBLEM-SOLVE)

Source: John Eldred, Transition I Associates, Ambler, Pa. Reproduced with permission.

Pick an issue or problem that you have to address — one that will involve at least the potential for conflict. Of the key stakeholders, pick one with whom you have a solid, even good, relationship and who is both an ally (or, at worst, an opponent) and is at least motivated (if not motivated and competent) to hard-problem-solve. Seriously consider asking for help in changing the way you negotiate. Perhaps share this chapter with him or her, and use it as a way to begin the conversation about changing.

Pay attention to what happens. Critique yourself. Invite the insights of others. Slowly, move to attempting hard problem solving in less friendly environs. Take your time. Learning the skill of hard problem solving will not convert your life into one large sea of tranquillity. It will, if mastered, help you negotiate more inspired agreements in less time for the benefit of more people than you could otherwise have effected. Learning to do that takes time. Give yourself a full chance to accomplish that learning. You and your stakeholders deserve no less.

A Note on Leadership

We are all barraged by a multitude of forces. We are barraged by people, events, and information. Worst of all, we are barraged by "circumstances beyond our control." The magnitude of such circumstances could (and occasionally does) cause us to throw in the towel and declare "No more." At times, the ground itself seems to be shifting.

The reality of increasingly complex and intertwined forces impinging on us is externally and internally verifiable. It is the way things are today. To ignore that reality is to court danger. Nonetheless, a greater danger exists: willed paralysis. Willed paralysis follows from the decision, conscious or unconscious, that our efforts are useless. They are not.

What you do matters for at least three reasons. First, the people reading this chapter have the distinct privilege of having a greater part of the world under more of their influence than do at least 95 percent of humanity. It often does not feel that way, but your position alone gives you more opportunity than most other people you know to affect how a part of the world looks and feels. You do not control it, but you certainly influence what your people do and how they feel about what they do. Second, your position means that you have a better chance of pushing back against the world outside your unit than do others. If you do not push back, then who will?

Third, each time someone wills paralysis on himself or herself the disease spreads, making increasing paralysis more likely.

Leadership means identifying a purpose and pursuing that purpose through one's own actions. The purpose can be grand in scale or it can be as circumscribed as changing the tenor of a single work relationship or the culture of one meeting. Approaching negotiation as problem solving can serve such purposes well. Its use involves a risk, frequently personal in nature, but then taking personal risk is part of what makes leaders leaders.

References

Block, P. *The Empowered Manager: Positive Political Skills at Work.* San Francisco: Jossey-Bass, 1987.

Fisher, R., and Ury, W. *Getting to Yes: Negotiating Agreement Without Giving In.* Boston: Houghton Mifflin, 1981.

Freeman, R. E. *Strategic Management.* Boston: Pitman, 1984.

Raiffa, H. *The Art and Science of Negotiation.* Cambridge, Mass.: Belknap Press, 1982.

Shea, G. "The Study of Bargaining and Conflict Behavior: Broadening the Conceptual Arena." *Journal of Conflict Resolution,* 1980, *24* (4), 706–741.

Walton, R. *Managing Conflict: Interpersonal Dialogue and Third-Party Roles.* (2nd ed.) Reading, Mass.: Addison-Wesley, 1987.

Index